The Nurse-Client Relationship in Mental Health Nursing

WORKBOOK GUIDES TO UNDERSTANDING AND MANAGEMENT

Second Edition

JANET A. SIMMONS, R.N., M.S., M.Ed.

Assistant Professor of Nursing,
Fitchburg State College,
Fitchburg, Massachusetts

1976   W. B. SAUNDERS COMPANY / Philadelphia / London / Toronto

W. B. Saunders Company: West Washington Square
Philadelphia, Pa.   19105

1 St. Anne's Road
Eastbourne, East Sussex BN21 3UN, England

833 Oxford Street
Toronto, M8Z 5T9, Canada

Library of Congress Cataloging in Publication Data

Simmons, Janet A
        The nurse-client relationship in mental health nursing.

        Bibliography: p.
        1. Psychiatric nursing. 2. Nurse and patient. I. Title. [DNLM: 1. Nurse-
patient relations. 2. Psychiatric nursing. WY160 S592n]
RC440.S49   1976   610.73'68   75-40639
ISBN 0-7216-8286-3

The Nurse-Client Relationship in Psychiatric Nursing   ISBN   0-7216-8286-3

Last digit is the print number: 9   8   7   6   5   4   3   2   1

To My Husband
Donald

PREFACE

This workbook has been designed to guide the nurse as she attempts to establish a therapeutic relationship with a person experiencing emotional difficulty in dealing with stress. Some theoretical material has been included as a brief introduction to each guide solely for the purpose of acquainting the nurse with the general theme to be explored. The student will need adequate textbooks to supply the theoretical background necessary to work with the client.

The author believes that the prime factor involved in any relationship is the establishment of mutual trust. The major task of the nurse in any nursing situation is to gain the confidence of the client so that she may successfully carry out whatever nursing function she is attempting, realizing that without this trust and acceptance she is likely to meet failure.

The attempt by the nurse to establish a basis for trust with a person under serious stress is intricate, complex, and time-consuming. However, trust must be established before she can meet her major nursing objective of encouraging the client to develop adaptive behavior or to exchange maladaptive behavior for that which will help him adjust constructively to his life situation.

The assumption is made that previous to the psychiatric–mental health nursing experience, the student has acquired a general knowledge in the areas of psychology, sociology, human growth and development, and interpersonal relations. It is also assumed that the student has texts available for the study of the dynamics of psychopathology.

The workbook is also based on the premise that the human individual functions best on an interdependent level and

v

that knowledge of the elements occurring in human relationships improves his ability to function at that level. Furthermore, at some period in his life, each individual experiences periods of stress during which the assistance of another person, while not necessarily required, will be of value, particularly when the assistance is offered on a knowledgeable rather than intuitive basis. Therefore, the relationships that occur between two people are of prime importance.

There are certain elements common to all relationships, whether between two "normal," well-adapted, mentally healthy individuals, or with the diagnosed psychotic or neurotic individual, or with an individual experiencing transient stress.

The workbook, therefore, serves as a guide to the understanding of those elements which will assist the student to develop healthy relationships with all individuals, no matter what their physical or psychological state of health or their relationship to her. The various guides are intended to help the student observe, evaluate, and eventually intervene, if necessary, in the events that take place. While the workbook focuses on the professional relationship in nursing, particularly the nursing of those experiencing emotional stress, it is the author's belief that all relationships are based on the elements herein described.

One of the basic understandings to be acquired in nursing the individual experiencing stress is the awareness of the impact one person has on another in any mutual relationship. Therefore, material has been included in the guides to help the student assess not only the effect that she has on the client but also the effect that the client has on her. The opportunity offered to assess and modify her own behavior hopefully will help the student in other nursing situations.

The relationship between the client and the nurse is a fluctuating, variable process. Therefore, rather than attempt merely to follow the sequence of this workbook, the student will need to be aware of its entire contents early in her experience so that she may complete the various sections as the client presents the material. For example, she may observe nonverbal behavior before she has verbally communicated with her client. She will then be able to use the guide related to nonverbal behavior which is presented later in the workbook.

The instructor may prefer to review the workbook at periodic intervals with the student in order to help the student validate her observations and behavior and to correct distortions which result from the personal bias of the student. The instructor's task of guiding the student is made easier by the fact that the student will be presenting her material in an orderly manner with some understanding of its meaning. However, the problem of controlling distortion in the student's observations, evaluations, and interventions will still depend in some part on the guidance of the instructor.

It is suggested that accurate recordings of the observations, events, and communications that occur in the relationship be maintained by the student so that she may obtain the material for the workbook. The author believes that the guides do not replace the necessity of maintaining recordings but rather help the student to organize data, so that she may eventually have an integrated picture of the elusive being who is her client.

The final evaluation included at the end of the workbook is designed to summarize major events that occurred during the nurse-client relationship. From this summary, the student may acquire a more specific knowledge of the importance and significance of what originally appeared to be isolated events and of their effect on the entire relationship. Recognition of her own progress in developing those skills and understandings necessary to the practice of psychiatric-mental health nursing will be more valid when viewed in the perspective of the entire experience rather than the limited picture obtained by isolating a few significant events.

Sincere gratitude is extended to the student nurses who were involved in the initial phases of testing the guides in the first edition of this workbook and in the present revision, as well as to all those whose encouragement and advice were invaluable in helping me to complete the task. A special debt is acknowledged to the author's mother, Mrs. George Martin, and to the author's daughter, Anna Mae Richards, for their endless hours of typing.

JANET A. SIMMONS

USE OF GUIDES

The guides in this workbook are designed for use by a nurse who is attempting to provide guidance and care for an individual experiencing emotional stress so that he may develop a positive, problem-solving approach to his stress.

A problem-solving approach is utilized to help the nurse plan and develop a course of action. The guides in Part I are directed toward helping the nurse determine what she needs to know, how she may acquire it, and then how to categorize her data. The task is complicated by the fact that while she is collecting data, she is at the same time attempting to perform in a therapeutic manner. She may be meeting immediate needs before she has collected sufficient data to develop a plan of care. As a result, some of the items in the guides in Part I are designed to direct the student toward meeting short-term goals as well as to establish the basis for her nursing care plan. The Guide for Communication exemplifies this problem. As the nurse collects data and observes the client's ability to communicate, she may purposefully or inadvertently help him to improve his skill. The process of collecting data then serves as the vehicle by which the client is helped to learn adaptive behavior.

The guides in Part II are to help the nurse assemble her observations in such a way that she is able to see the behavioral pattern of her client in total as he functions in his environment rather than as a series of isolated characteristics. On the basis of her organized observations and interpretations, she is directed toward developing a nursing care plan on a long-range, individualized basis rather than on the basis of the short-term, nonspecific goals utilized before sufficient data were available.

The guides in Part III direct the nurse as she attempts to encourage the development of adaptive behavior on the part of the client.

The final guide in Part IV focuses the attention of the nurse on the overall picture of the entire relationship. The emphasis is placed specifically on changes that occurred, what brought them about, and what hindered progress.

Items are included in all of the guides to help the nurse observe and evaluate her own behavior, its effect on others, and its effect on the therapeutic process.

If the nurse is using the workbook without the help of an instructor, its chief use will be to serve as a means of indicating the kind of information she needs and the use she will make of her data once she has organized it. It may also help her to avoid some common pitfalls that occur when one attempts to establish a therapeutic rather than a social relationship. It would be advisable for her to check her observations and interpretations regularly with another person in order to uncover her own bias.

When the nurse works with an instructor, the workbook may be used to indicate areas in which the nurse needs help. Many of the items may suggest a basis for a nursing conference if the instructor finds an area of difficulty common to many nurses. The author has found that a frequent review of her students' workbooks has given a reasonably accurate picture of events which occur in the nurse-client relationship but which the student may not present in conference because she forgets various details or thinks that certain events are not significant enough to warrant comment.

Experience with the first edition of the workbook indicated to the author that answers to the questions in the guides will vary according to the student's educational and experiential background. For example, the question "Are you afraid of your client?" may be answered "No" by a very unsophisticated student, whereas the student with more depth of background may respond "Yes. The client may react to a homosexual panic by striking me." The workbook, therefore, is applicable to varying levels of nursing students but responses will vary.

CONTENTS

PART I

OBSERVATION AND COLLECTION OF DATA

CHAPTER 1

Orientation

The first meeting between nurse and client usually produces anxiety for both participants. It is a time of assessment and commitment—assessment of each other and the dangers involved, and commitment to each other with the prospect of closeness, intimacy, and separation. Courage to face the emotional storms that are inevitable, patience to continue the search for progress, and hope that the present pain and suffering will be alleviated underlie the agreement that is made.

The orientation period provides an opportunity for both nurse and client to acquire certain facts about each other, to make observations concerning the other's behavior, and to lay the foundation for a working, therapeutic relationship. Both nurse and client will use past knowledge gained from other interpersonal contacts. From the beginning, the nurse seeks to establish a professional, rather than a social, relationship. If this is the first experience the client has had with such a relationship, the nurse will need to explain carefully, and more than once, the terms of the contract she and the client are making. Having established the terms under which she and the client will meet and work, she must abide by them scrupulously, expecting the client to do likewise to the best of his ability.

The client may attempt to place the relationship on a social rather than a professional basis. Questions concerning the personal life of the nurse are common. The nurse will need to decide whether or not the answers to such questions will serve a professional purpose. The client, in order to establish realistic facts about the nurse as a person, may need to know her approximate age, whether she is married, and if she has a family. However, knowledge of the nurse's activities the previous evening scarcely seems relevant to a working relationship.

The client needs to know the status and role of the nurse and her reasons for attempting to establish a relationship with him. The nurse's activity during the orientation period may cause the client to expect that her behavior during subsequent interactions will be similar. Therefore, if she asks many questions instead of simply listening to the client, he may expect her to continue to do so. The nurse needs to make clear that the time when she is with the client is for him to talk about what he wishes, or to remain quiet if he wishes. Her contribution to the relationship is the fact that she is present to listen and to help if she can.

In any contract, certain terms are stipulated. The nurse and the client agree on a time and place of meeting, the duration of each meeting, and a termination date. The nurse explains her purposes and describes any activities, such as making recordings, that will occur. She also explains how the recordings will be used. The client must agree to the terms of the contract. The nurse stipulates that the interaction between herself and the client and any information divulged in their meetings are confidential. To maintain confidentiality, the nurse uses the client's initial rather than his name on her recordings, and takes care to keep the recordings in her possession. However, if students meet in conference groups to discuss their recordings, no matter how careful a student is to conceal the name of the client there is a possibility that his identity will become known. Therefore, the entire conference group must be bound by the contract.

Although the student emphasizes that she will not reveal to others what is told to her in confidence, she may be faced with a dilemma if the client tells her he is about to harm himself or someone else, leave a hospital without permission, or break the law in some way. If she reveals the information, she will break the contract and destroy the client's trust. However, if she remains silent, the client may commit suicide or otherwise cause harm. The student's professional obligation is to protect the client. Therefore, to avoid such a dilemma, the student, when making the contract, must indicate that information of such a nature will be revealed to the doctor or other responsible personnel. The nurse may state that she will ask the client to tell the doctor himself and will accompany the client if he needs such support. If the client states that he will not consult his psychiatrist, then the nurse indicates that she will convey the necessary information herself. She assures the client, however, that before doing so, she will tell the client what she proposes doing. In this way, the client will be assured that his confidence will not be betrayed and, in fact, he will not reveal anything he does not wish known.

The nurse also has a responsibility to acquaint other professionals responsible for her client's care with the progress of the relationship between herself and the client. She may do so without breaking confidentiality by describing events in broad terms but omitting specific details. For example, she may state that the client is having difficulty in initiating activities, without describing the actual activity or the client's abortive attempts at initiation. The fact that the nurse will make such a report as well as what she actually says to other professional personnel is to be shared with the client.

PRE-ORIENTATION GUIDE

Answer the following questions before your initial orientation interaction with a client.

1. List information you need about your client before beginning the interview.

Where can you obtain this information?

Why do you need it?

2. List information your client will need about you when he is first introduced to you.

Why will he need this information?

3. List information your client will not need about you.

Why will he not need the information you listed?

If your client asks for information that he does not need or that you do not wish to tell him, what will you say?

GUIDE FOR ORIENTATION

Answer the following questions after you have made the contract.

Information about the Client

1. Age   Sex   Marital Status

   Number of Children

   Other Family Members

   Occupations: Present

                 Past

   Education

2. Physical Health

   Height   Weight

   Presence of Physical Illness

   Presence of Deformity

Past Physical Illnesses

3. Mental Health

Diagnosis   I.Q.

Past History

4. Reason for referral:

Information about You

1. List information you volunteered about yourself. State your reasons for giving it. What was the client's response to the information?

2. List questions the client asked about you and the number of times he sought the same information. List your answers to the questions and state your reasons for your answers. Do you think your answers were appropriate to the therapeutic situation? If not, how would you change them?

Information about the Interview

1. What did you say about the purpose of the interview? What was the client's response?

2. What arrangements did you make as to time, place, and length of each meeting? What was the client's response?

3. Describe briefly the setting selected for your meetings.

   1. Provision for privacy

   2. Degree of isolation

   3. Provisions for physical comfort

   4. Noise level

4. Are you comfortable in this setting? Explain your answer.

5. Describe any changes in the setting that you would like to make and state your reasons for the changes and the plans you are making to bring about the change.

6. What did you say about the ultimate termination? What was the client's response?

INSTRUCTOR'S COMMENTS

CHAPTER 2

Observation of Anxiety

Fear and anxiety are usually differentiated in terms of their object. Fear is caused by a readily identified, usually dangerous object or situation. The cause of anxiety is not readily apparent, may relate as much to past experiences as present, and is usually a diffuse feeling of emotional discomfort. One is afraid *of* but anxious *about* something. Removal of the dangerous object removes the fear. However, removal of anxiety is much more difficult. First, the reason for the anxiety needs to be identified. Psychoanalysis is required at times to identify the source of anxiety.

Frequently fear and anxiety occur simultaneously and are related to the same object. One may be both afraid and anxious about crossing a busy street—afraid of the rush of traffic and anxious about crossing any street, even when there is no traffic. In the first instance, the traffic is a real and present danger. One is justifiably afraid. The fear may be removed when the traffic stops or if one crosses the street with the help of a pedestrian traffic light. In the second instance, the reason for the anxiety is unknown. Crossing the street represents a symbol or displacement of a feeling of terror from some unknown object to the act of crossing the street. The choice of symbol for the feeling of anxiety bears a relationship to the cause but may be so well repressed that it is difficult to determine.

Both fear and anxiety are caused by a threat as perceived by the individual. The threat may be that of pain, discomfort, or an assault on the self-image. Observable causes, therefore, are unique to the individual. An object that threatens the self-image of one individual is perceived as innocuous by another.

Anxiety is assumed by some authors to be related to the birth experience, which is both painful and life-threatening. Subsequent experiences which are perceived as painful or life-threatening reactivate the original, or primal, anxiety. Numbers of anxiety-provoking experiences, in which the anxiety is not completely resolved but leaves a residue of feeling, may produce a state of chronic anxiety. The individual wakens in the morning with a diffuse feeling that "something is wrong" but cannot pinpoint any specific cause. This type of anxiety is called free-floating. Anxiety related to causes other than the birth experience is referred to as secondary.

11

Anxiety tends to be contagious. An experience similar to an anxiety-provoking past experience will evoke anxiety based on the similarity even when the likeness is minute. Furthermore, the perception of danger by one individual may cause anxiety in another, although the second individual perceives only the anxiety of the first and not any specific threat.

The signs and symptoms of anxiety are both physical and psychological manifestations which prepare the individual for fight or flight. The most obvious physical signs are those related to muscular tension in which facial muscles may be observed to tighten or twitch, hands or feet will shake, and the individual will fidget or pace. Pallor or flushing of the face accompanied by diaphoresis may be present. The pupils of the eyes may dilate widely. Temperature and blood pressure are elevated; vomiting, diarrhea, and frequent urination may appear depending on the severity of the perceived danger and the ability of the individual to cope with anxiety.

The most important psychological manifestation of anxiety is the effect on the individual's ability to perceive accurately and without distortion. Four levels of anxiety may be identified, ranging from mild to moderate to severe to panic. In mild anxiety the individual's attention is diffuse and unfocused. He is more or less in a state of rest, paying attention to nothing in particular but aware of his environment and alert enough to identify any signs of threat. Physically there are no observable signs of tension. In moderate anxiety, some change has occurred to alert the individual to some need to act. The need to act represents a possible threat. At this point, muscles begin to tense, mild diaphoresis may occur, and the attention becomes focused directly upon the anxiety-producing object. Other stimuli in the environment tend to be tuned out. The individual perceives with a great deal of accuracy and with minimal distortion.

If the anxiety increases from moderate to severe, physical manifestations markedly increase, the most obvious being trembling and excessive motor activity, widely dilated pupils, and excessive diaphoresis. Of great importance at this level is the effect on attention which now, because of the perception of an extreme danger, cannot focus on the threat itself but turns aside to focus on some other stimulus of a less threatening nature. The individual at this point, then, has shifted his focus of attention so that he not only perceives inaccurately and incompletely but tends to distort what he does see.

In the most severe level of anxiety, one which seldom occurs and is usually of short duration, a state of panic ensues which is characterized by a total lack of focus. The individual is unable to react in other than an apparently purposeless running or thrashing about, unresponsive to his environment and people in it. His attention is unfocused and cannot be channeled or guided until the panic has subsided. Unrelieved panic can result in death. Usually the physical behavior is so bizarre and uncontrollable that controls are enforced by others, including the use of physical restraint. The restraint and presence of others usually provides enough evidence that help is available to relieve the anxiety and move it from the panic level to the severe level which, while uncomfortable, is not life-threatening.

The assessment of the level of anxiety both in herself and in the client is of prime importance to the nurse in planning her care. Anxiety as defined here is not necessarily unpleasant or undesirable. Unless there is a moderate degree of anxiety, the process of learning is seriously handicapped. Learning requires a focusing of attention on the subject at hand with accurate and undistorted perception. The nurse must, therefore, induce a moderate degree of anxiety in both herself and the client if their relationship is to be one in which learning takes place. Occasionally, severe anxiety will occur either in the nurse or the client, in the nurse as a result of a threat to her nursing ability by the client, or in the client as emotions from past experiences are reactivated or if present events are perceived as threatening. The nurse needs to be aware that the severe level of anxiety can be tolerated for a period of time but that eventually it must be reduced to a moderate level for learning to occur. The nurse should never leave the client at the severe level of anxiety.

Observation of physical signs and symptoms in the orientation phase of the one-to-one relationship will help the nurse identify the level of anxiety in herself and in the client. While she is collecting data, she will not wish to encourage severe anxiety and, if she sees it occurring, will attempt to reduce the degree. Once a nursing care plan has been developed, the nurse may wish to introduce anxiety-provoking material or situations which will produce severe anxiety. However, by this point in the relationship a degree of trust and comfort between nurse and client will have been established that will allow the maintenance of a greater anxiety level for a period of time following which the level may be reduced.

The experience and knowledge gained during the period of severe anxiety may then be examined during a period of moderate anxiety so that distortions may be evaluated and learning may occur. As an example, a nurse working with a client who is terrified of entering a crowded supermarket will develop the relationship initially to a point where the client is at ease with her and believes that the nurse can and will help him if need be. When this point is reached, nurse and client together may decide to enter the market. The client, as he approaches and enters the market, will very likely experience a severe level of anxiety but, knowing help is available in the presence of the nurse, may be able to tolerate the experience. The nurse, too, will likely experience an increase in her own anxiety, knowing that she may be required to perform quickly and publicly in a tense situation. Once the nurse and the client leave the market, their anxiety levels will decrease and together they may evaluate what happened, combine their observations in order to correct distortions and add missing details, identify helpful activities, and plan a second visit to the supermarket.

Anxiety is an uncomfortable feeling that results from a threat. To protect himself from the discomfort of anxiety, the individual develops measures to avoid, disguise, or eliminate the threat. Such measures are usually called defense mechanisms or coping devices. The greater number of such measures available for use by the individual, the more ways he has to deal with the threat. If he has developed only a few protective measures, he will tend to function in a stereotyped, inflexible manner and will, therefore, be less able to cope with a threat. It is suggested that the nurse review in any general psychology book the descriptions of the various defensive maneuvers. Identification of the means by which the client deals with anxiety is necessary in order to determine the effectiveness of his adaptation to his environment and the need for nursing intervention.

GUIDE FOR OBSERVATION OF ANXIETY I

Directions: Items in this guide are related to observations made during the orientation phase of the one-to-one relationship. This begins with the initial contact and is concluded when the client indicates clear understanding and acceptance of the contract. Select material from your recordings during this period to complete the items.

1. List signs and symptoms of anxiety observed in the client during your initial greeting and before indicating your desire to initiate a nurse-client relationship.

    a. Physical   b. Psychological

2. Identify the level of anxiety indicated by your response to the previous question. Include any apparent reasons for the level of anxiety displayed by the client.

3. List signs and symptoms of anxiety that you experienced during your initial greeting.

    a. Physical   b. Psychological

4.   Identify your level of anxiety during the period described. Include reasons for your level of anxiety and describe any outward manifestation of your anxiety.

5.   Describe any response by the client that you think may have resulted from his observation of your anxiety.

6.   Describe signs and symptoms of anxiety observed in the client as you proposed the terms of the contract.

     a.   Physical   b.   Psychological

7.   Identify the level of anxiety indicated by the client as the terms of the contract were stated. Include any marked response to a specific item in the contract.

8. Describe the effect of the anxiety level reached on the client's ability to understand the terms of the contract. Include the number of times you found it necessary to repeat the terms of the contract.

9. State items in the contract that the client questioned or failed to meet at subsequent meetings as a result of misunderstanding.

10. Identify your level of anxiety as you proposed the contract. Include any difficulty you had in stating a specific item and the apparent reasons for your anxiety level.

11. Describe the effects of your anxiety level on your ability to state the contract and to observe the client's response.

12.   Identify the level of anxiety indicated by your client as you prepared to terminate the meeting. Include any change in the signs and symptoms observed.

13.   Identify your level of anxiety as you terminated the meeting. Describe your behavior and feelings immediately after leaving the client.

14.   Identify any defense mechanism you observed the client use. Include a description of the event, of the behavior that you identify as defensive, and of the result of the defensive mechanism.

15.   Identify any defensive mechanism you used. Indicate the reason for using the defense, its efficiency in reducing your anxiety, and its possible effect on the proposed one-to-one relationship.

GUIDE FOR OBSERVATION OF ANXIETY II

Directions: Items in this guide are related to those observations made during the orientation phase after the terms of the contract have been accepted and before the statement of the major problem (the nursing care plan) is made. These observations refer to that part of the relationship during which trust and acceptance are being developed and the nurse collects data needed for the actual care plan. Answer the following items from material in your recordings and your observations.

1. Describe the level of anxiety you observe in your client during the meeting which takes place immediately after that one in which the client accepted the terms of the contract. Indicate the basis of your assessment of the anxiety level.

2. Describe your own anxiety level during the meeting indicated in the previous question. State the reasons for your level of anxiety.

3. Describe any events that occurred during the orientation period, within or outside of the nurse-client relationship, that caused an increase in his anxiety. Include the client's response and any intervention on your part.

4. Describe any communication concerning himself, other people, or the milieu that produced an increase in anxiety. Include the basis for your assessment.

5. Describe the chief defenses against anxiety that you observed during this period. Include the cause of the anxiety, the identification of defense mechanisms used, behavior manifested, results of the defenses, and any intervention on your part.

GUIDE FOR OBSERVATION OF ANXIETY III

Directions: Items in this guide are related to observations made during the working phase of the relationship. The working phase begins immediately after the client accepts the statement of his major problem and is concluded after the nursing care plan has been implemented, when the client is about to consider the termination of the relationship. Select material from your recordings during this period to complete the items.

1. List the defense mechanisms that you have observed the client using as his problem was stated and the care plan implemented.

2. From the preceding list, select two defenses that occur with the greatest frequency. Describe on the opposite page the events that take place that apparently cause the client to use the defenses, and evaluate the efficiency of the defenses in reducing anxiety and in producing a long-range solution to the removal or reduction of the threat.

3. Describe meetings during which the client's anxiety remained at the mild level. Include reasons for anxiety being at this level.

4. Describe any intervention on your part to maintain the client at the mild level of anxiety or to move the client to the moderate level of anxiety. State your reasons for the intervention and evaluate the result. Suggest any changes for future interventions.

5. Describe experiences in which the client's level of anxiety moved from moderate to severe. Include the reasons for the move, the length of time the client remained at a severe level, and the indications you had that the client was at the severe level.

Defense	Description	Increase or Decrease of Anxiety	Long-range Result
1.			
2.			

6.   From one of the preceding experiences, describe the client's return to a moderate or mild level of anxiety. Include the reasons for the change and indications of the change.

7.   Evaluate the results of the experience with severe anxiety in respect to the client's ability to tolerate increasing amounts of anxiety.

8.   Evaluate the effect of severe anxiety in assisting the client to develop a different approach to the anxiety-producing situation.

9.   Describe your level of anxiety during one of the episodes in which the client was at the severe level of anxiety. Include the signs and symptoms of which you were aware and any signs that you think the client recognized. What means did you use to keep your anxiety manageable and how successful were you? What was the effect of your anxiety on your attempts at intervention with the client?

10. Describe any changes in the client that have occurred during this entire working phase in relation to the following:

    a. Number of defense mechanisms used.

    b. Appearance of new defenses.

    c. Frequency with which defenses were used.

    d. Effectiveness of defenses used.

    e. Amount of severe anxiety generated.

    f. Precipitating causes of any increase in anxiety.

    g. Duration of periods of mild anxiety.

    h. Duration of periods of moderate anxiety.

    i. Duration of periods of severe anxiety.

11. Describe any changes in your level of anxiety. What moves your anxiety from moderate to severe?

GUIDE FOR OBSERVATION OF ANXIETY IV

Directions: Items in this guide are related to observations made during the terminal phase of the relationship. The terminal phase is that period following the implementation of the plan of care when the nurse and client are preparing to close the relationship. Select material from your recordings during this period to complete the items.

1. List signs and symptoms of anxiety that occurred when you made a statement that termination was imminent.

2. Compare the preceding indications of anxiety with the response the client made when you stated the termination date during the setting of the contract in relation to the following:

	Orientation Period	Terminal Period
Level		
Duration		
Defense		
Result		

3. Describe your anxiety level when you stated termination was imminent. State the apparent causes for your level of anxiety.

4. Describe any intervention on your part to increase or decrease the level of anxiety generated in the client in response to termination. Include the reason for and the results of your intervention and suggest changes needed.

5. Describe any defenses used by the client to assist him with termination. Evaluate them as to whether they are adaptive or maladaptive.

6. Describe any intervention on your part to encourage adaptive measures or discourage maladaptive defenses that occurred in your client in response to termination. Include the results of your intervention.

7. Describe any attempt on your part to use adaptive or maladaptive measures to deal with termination. Include the results of your attempt.

8. Describe the level of anxiety observed in your client as you terminated your last meeting. How accurate was your observation?

INSTRUCTOR'S COMMENTS

CHAPTER 3

Communication Skills

To assess the needs of her client, the nurse must not only use her powers of observation but must also develop the ability to communicate in such a way that she understands what her client says, her client understands what she says, and the health team comprehends what both are saying.

Communication involves a sender, a message, and a receiver. The cycle may be considered effective when the message is understood by the receiver in the approximate manner that the sender intended. The message may be considered ineffective when the receiver derives a meaning other than that intended by the sender.

In the nursing situation, the client and nurse are both viewed alternately as sender and receiver. The client-sender relays a message to the nurse-receiver who, in turn, becomes a sender as she responds to the client or carries his message to other members of the health team. In this complex cycle, many factors influence the accuracy of the message conveyed. In assessing client needs, the nurse needs to be aware of the factors that either facilitate or detract from communication as it is sent or received.

In actual practice, verbal communication does not take place without nonverbal communication occurring simultaneously. In fact, there are many instances in nursing practice in which the only form of communication is nonverbal. Many times, also, nonverbal communication is at variance with verbal communication.

This guide will deal specifically with verbal communication as a separate entity. A subsequent guide will then consider nonverbal communication, although it must be emphasized that the division is purely academic.

Factors That Affect or Distort Communication. In assessing communication needs, the nurse must be aware of those factors that influence the sender, those that affect the message itself, and those that influence the receiver.

Some factors influencing the sender relate to the mechanical ability to send or produce sound: lack of dentition, mouth, nose, or throat anomalies or disease, or disease processes such as aphasia.

Another factor is motivation. Many times because of embarrassment, fear, or personal motives, the sender may decide to conceal or distort information. The client who has a purulent vaginal discharge may complain of not being allowed to bathe frequently, rather than explaining that she has an irritating discharge that is temporarily relieved by a bath. She may be embarrassed to explain something of a personal nature, she may fear a vaginal examination or the possibility of a serious illness, or she may view the discharge as punishment for sin and something to be endured silently. Likewise, the nurse who must explain the recordings of the nurse-client interactions to the client may fear that such information will cause the client to reject the proposed nurse-client relationship. Therefore, she may "forget" to mention the recordings or may describe them so hurriedly that their necessity and importance are minimized to the point that the client does not understand their significance or even why they must be maintained by the student.

The schizophrenic client who uses a system of paleologic, that is, a primitive logic different from the more mature logic of the nurse, may communicate by inventing his own words, or neologisms, words that have no meaning for anyone other than himself.* He also may assign the same meaning to words that merely sound alike or use them because he enjoys pronouncing repetitious sounds. The following is an example of such an association, which is usually referred to as a clang association:

> Where is the hare?
> Here is the hare (hair).
> Hair on my head, wed, bed.

The client may also show a disturbance in his ability to communicate understandably because he is using a loose association of words based on faulty identification. The client who identifies himself as Napoleon may be attempting to say that he is French, or that he is a very short man, or that he possesses tremendous power. Without clarification, the nurse is unable to understand such a communication. The following has been selected from a recording made by a student to illustrate the manner in which a client constructs a loose association:

> Adam and atom. It's a funny thing they're the same. Just change one letter. Adam was first and everything is made of atoms. Everyone is related because of Adam and Eve and everything is made up of atoms.

The client may condense either words or sentences so that he produces what is commonly called a "word salad." Thus the sentence, "The way to the movies is through the tunnel," may be produced as "Way to move tun." Such messages may convey no meaning to the nurse.

The nurse may communicate by using abstract terminology and symbolisms characterized by figures of speech such as the metaphor. The mentally ill client understands and uses concrete rather than abstract terminology. When the average person says "The wolf is at the door," he means that he is in a desperate financial state. In contrast, when the mentally ill person says "The wolf is at the door," he probably means the statement literally—that a wolf of the four-legged variety is visible.

---

*For a more detailed description of the use of paleologic by the schizophrenic patient, the student is advised to refer to "Interpretation of Schizophrenia" by Silvano Ariete, published by Robert Brunner, Inc., New York, 1955.

Children make similar literal interpretations. Once at a family gathering the comment was made that the teen-age son was "growing out of his clothes." Attention was suddenly focused on the five year old who was watching in amazement apparently expecting the growth phenomenon to occur before his very eyes. Many such expressions, of which we are generally unaware, are a part of everyday speech. The nurse, as a communication sender, must carefully examine her own speech to delete abstractions that may be misinterpreted by the client.

The communication cycle may also be disrupted by factors within the message itself. The variety of meanings assigned or conveyed in one word or in a phrase may result in distortion. When I say "She was fast," my meaning is not clear because I have used an indefinite word, she, which may refer to a boat that is tied, a car that travels rapidly, or a person of questionable morals.

Language barriers, difficulties in enunciation, and inappropriate terminology, added to background noises, distractions, and confusion, adversely affect the message.

The receiver completes the communication cycle. Communication failure at this point may be caused by the physical inability of the receiver to hear. Hearing only bits and pieces of the message, he may invent the rest at his pleasure with or without a drastic change in meaning.

What the client hears is also affected by the attention or selective inattention which he affords the message. He may not want to hear about the subject being discussed, or he may hear only those parts which he wants to hear. This is like the teen-ager who has been granted permission to use the family car if he provides the gas but hears only the pleasant part of the message and leaves the gas tank empty. When the subject matter is particularly stressful, the nurse may suspect that the client will hear only a part of her message. The maintenance of recordings may produce so much anxiety for the paranoid client that, because of selective inattention, he will not hear all of the nurse's explanation about the use of recordings and will distort that which he does hear.

The understanding of the person receiving the message may be limited by his educational background or by his intellectual ability to comprehend the message as it is conveyed.

As was mentioned earlier, the receiver may misinterpret the message sent because he is unable to understand abstract terminology. He will also interpret the message in the context of past experiences. The nurse may say, "Let's go for a walk," with the intent of spending a pleasant hour outside in the fresh air. The client, however, may remember that on a former occasion when a nurse said, "Let's go for a walk," he was taken to another ward to receive electric shock treatment. Because of his earlier, unfortunate experience, he may refuse vigorously what the nurse innocently offered as a pleasant excursion. In this instance, the client's refusal relays a message of hostility to the nurse, which she, in turn, may not understand because she, as a receiver, interprets his response as she has others like it in the past. To prevent such a complete breakdown of the communication cycle, the nurse must assume responsibility for clarifying the messages sent and the understanding gained.

The communication cycle is the means used by the individual to establish and validate the reality of the environment. The mentally ill client who may have retreated from a commonly accepted reality is in need of the nurse's ability to present reality factors as clearly and as free from distortion as she is able. The opportunities for consensual validation by the client may be limited by his withdrawal and his lack of skill in developing and tolerating interpersonal relations. By correcting some of the unreality that keeps the client isolated, the nurse may serve as the bridge that helps him to reach out toward others and toward his environment.

By persistently encouraging the client to clarify, explain, and describe events which are significant to him, the nurse may gradually help him to abandon the use of paleologic. In helping him to attempt to describe his meanings so that she may understand him, she will force him to identify and conceptualize in such a way that loose associations are avoided. The following example selected from a recording of a nurse-client interaction illustrates an attempt by a student to encourage the client to describe his meanings more clearly.

Client: "I'm thinking of the number 7."
Nurse: "What does the number 7 mean to you?"
Client: "Well, they say we have six senses. Maybe we have seven."
Nurse: "Go on."
Client: "Well, it's like dollars and cents. Dollars are worth more than cents. It is written in the Lord's prayer."
Nurse: "What is written in the Lord's Prayer?"
Client: "Sense."

The nurse, too, in order to be sure that her communications are being received in the same context that she sends them will need to develop a means of assessing her effectiveness. Cues to the client's understanding of her message may be derived from his verbal or nonverbal responses. The maintenance of reasonably accurate and complete recordings of the nurse-client interaction, which may be checked by the student and her instructor, will help the student to become aware of any difficulties she might have in transmitting communications accurately and in receiving the client's responses without undue distortion.

Cognitive and Affective Modes of Communication. The nurse, as a therapeutic agent, has a responsibility to identify cue words used by the client that indicate some of the underlying meaning and emotions being conveyed. Cue words may be characterized as those in the cognitive domain and those in the affective domain. Cognitive words are those that indicate factual material. Affective words are those that indicate emotions. Cognitive words may arouse an affective response because they relate to past experiences which had an emotional component. Misinterpretation can occur in either domain. For example, on a cognitive level, it is a common experience to become lost when attempting to follow directions to a strange place, the misinterpretation arising either in the sender, the receiver, or both. Similarly, in the affective domain, the sender may say that he dislikes something when, in fact, he means he is afraid of that something. The previous comment made by the nurse to the client about going for a walk is an example of a message containing words in the cognitive domain but to which the client responded on an affective level.

When the nurse sends a message on the cognitive level, she needs to assess the client's understanding of her message. She may do this by asking the client to re-peat the message or by asking questions to determine his understanding. Similar-ly, when she receives a message in the cognitive domain, she needs to determine that she has interpreted the message correctly. She may do this by repeating to the client what she has understood and asking for verification. A common area for such misunderstandings to occur may be found during the setting of the terms of a contract, particularly in regard to time and place. Misunderstandings may result in client and nurse waiting for each other at different times in dif-ferent places.

Communication During the Phases of the Relationship. When the one-to-one relationship is in its beginning phase, the client tends to use many cognitive words, phrases, or themes. At times he produces a great deal of past and present history which seems to be affective in nature. For example, he may describe very painful relations with other people or very traumatic experiences at work. How-ever, he is actually recounting factual material. There will be some degree of emotion involved, but the nurse will discover that this emotion tends to be more superficial than that which will occur midway through the relationship.

Following the initial flurry in which so much material is presented, the client is likely to state that he has "nothing else to talk about." What he is indicating is that he has indeed produced a great deal of information but he has reached the end of the cognitive data. He is at the crossroads when, if he is to progress, he must stop intellectualizing and move into the affective domain, or the pre-working phase* of the relationship. During the working phase, affective data will be dom-inant. Cognitive data that occurs during this phase will be used to describe or em-phasize the affective data, and the cognitive data will definitely be subordinate.

Again, as the client moves into the terminal phase, there will be a re-surfacing of cognitive words and themes which will be directed toward future planning rather than toward past or present experiences. This final cognitive phase will be balanced with affective data occurring in depth and related both to the impending loss and impending insecurity and stress related to events planned for the future. This may be diagrammed as follows:

Beginning Phase	Working Phase	Termination
Cognitive Data* (past-present orientation)	**Affective Data** (in depth)	**Cognitive Data** (future planning)
Affective Data (superficial)	Cognitive Data (related solely to dominant)	**Affective Data** (in depth-related to loss and future planning)

*Boldface lettering indicates dominance of type of data

---

*Pre-working phase in this respect refers to the development of trust which immediately precedes the true working phase.

During the dominance of cognitive production, the nurse may identify one or two themes which keep recurring. The recurrence indicates that there is some affective material of importance connected to the recurring themes. If the client has difficulty in moving from the cognitive level to the affective level, the nurse can assist the client by referring to one of the recurring themes and suggesting that the client appears to have serious concerns in this area. By providing clarification and complete descriptions of these areas, the client may be able to identify the underlying effects and so move into the working phase of the relationship.

The nurse needs to be particularly attuned to words in the affective domain since they are most likely to give cues to areas of emotional concern for the client. Words such as "love" or "hate" or "sadness" indicate powerful emotions which need occur only once to alert the nurse. There are, however, other more subtle words which by the frequency of their occurrence indicate a possible concern. When the client's speech is liberally sprinkled with words such as "I will," "I won't," "Don't tell me," "I am," "Can I," "Maybe," "I wonder," "What do you think," the nurse receives a cue that the client may be experiencing difficulty in making decisions. His ability to assert himself or to make decisions may be so tenuous that it will not withstand questioning. Therefore, he may state "I will" or "I won't" and imply that he is not to be questioned. Conversely, he may be unable to say "I will" or "I won't" but must depend on the opinion of someone else. Therefore, he will say "maybe" or "I wonder," expecting verification from the listener.

The client may also make frequent use of the words "ought," "should," "must," "good," "bad," "right," or "wrong," giving the nurse the cue that he is likely to be functioning with an excessive amount of guilt. When the words "good" or "bad" refer to work performance rather than moral issues, the nurse may suspect feelings of inferiority.

The frequency with which affective words occur is a cue in itself to areas of emotional concern. The individual who is applying the words "love" and "hate" to the same object and practically in the same sentence, if not actually in the same sentence, is indicating ambivalence toward that object. When powerful words such as "love" and "hate" are used consistently or in place of milder terms such as "like" or "dislike," the client is likely to be one who has poor emotional control, who is at the mercy of violent emotional upheavals, and who is emotionally labile.

In contrast to the emotionally labile individual is the client who rarely uses an affective word. His lack of emotional expression indicates an apathy or a blunting of the affect that is "characteristic of" the schizophrenic.

When the nurse receives a cue that a possible emotional concern is being indicated, it is her responsibility to respond in such a way that the client is aware that she has recognized the cue and wishes to pursue the concern. Needless to say, it requires careful listening to identify cues. It also requires some skill to respond in such a way that the client will feel comfortable, or at least able, to consider painful concerns. There are techniques which will assist the nurse but caution must be exercised that the technique is adapted to the nurse's usual pattern of communicating and that a varied approach is used. If the client identifies the fact that the nurse is using a specific technique, he may decide that she is not being genuine and sincere but is simply following a textbook technique rather than being interested in him as a person.

The major aim of the nurse's response is to help the client describe fully what is bothering him. She, therefore, first indicates that she received the cue. This tells the client that she is actively listening and is interested. She then clarifies her understanding of the cue to avoid any misinterpretation. This also serves the purpose of helping the client examine and add to what he has already said. She then seeks greater clarification by asking for more details. At this point, she may move into actual intervention and her responses will be dictated by the therapeutic plan. The following is an example of an affective cue presented by a client and recognized and clarified by the nurse. The client then examines what he has said. The nurse responds by asking for greater clarification until a full description is evident.

Client: "I went to the movies last night but I hated the picture."
Nurse: "You say you 'hated' the picture. What about the picture did you hate?"
Client: "Well, I guess it wasn't really the picture. The auditorium was too hot."
Nurse: "You could not enjoy the movie because you were uncomfortable. The auditorium was too hot. What else made you uncomfortable?"
Client: "Too many people."

In this example, the nurse first recognized the cue she identified by repeating it to the client in his own words, "You hated the picture." Hate is the affective word. She then sought clarification by asking what it was the client hated. The client's response that the auditorium was too hot indicates that he is exploring and correcting what he has said. The nurse again responds to the affective statement, "too hot" but, instead of reflecting the exact words of the client as she had previously, varies her approach and reflects what she perceives to be the meaning of both of his statements, "You were uncomfortable." She then seeks further clarification of the situation by asking for more details in the question, "What else made you uncomfortable?" The client's response, "Too many people" is an indication of a serious problem, and at this point a therapeutic intervention might be considered.

In seeking clarification, note that in both instances the nurse asked a "what" question. If the nurse had asked why the client hated the picture, he might readily have answered "I don't know," because actually it was not the picture that was upsetting him. The nurse might also have asked "When did you go to the movies" and received the answer, "7:00 P.M." This question does not recognize the affective word "hate." It puts the communication on a cognitive level, thus leading the client away from an affective problem and subtly telling him that the nurse has not recognized the cue or is unwilling to talk about it. The nurse might also have said, "Do you usually feel uncomfortable when you go to the movies?" and received a "yes" or "no" response from the client. A leading question such as a "do you" or "don't you" gives the client the opportunity to answer in one word but does not provide for clarification or further description. The client, in fact, may simply tell the nurse what he thinks she wants to hear. In general, when seeking clarification, a "what" question will serve to open channels of exploration. "When" questions may be used at a later date if the time element has a bearing on the problem. It is also helpful when the "what" details have been established to find out who else is involved. In attempting to acquire more details, the nurse may reflect what she has been told, indicate what she does not understand or areas where she feels information is lacking, and then ask to be told the details that are missing. The phrases "I don't understand," "Please explain – – –," and "Tell me more about – – –" are most helpful in this respect.

In the early period of the nurse-client relationship, when the nurse is trying to improve both her skill and the client's skill in communication, she will have the opportunity to acquire data relative to the client's image of himself and of his environment, as well as data concerning the emotions he expresses and possible areas of maladaptive functioning. Such data will increase the nurse's understanding of her client, but it may not be appropriate at this point in the relationship to intervene in problems other than those related to the development of communication skills. Once a basis for trust has been established, the nurse may then intervene in a variety of problem areas. It seems advisable to categorize the data acquired so that it will be available for future use. Therefore, in the following communication guides, some items relate to the client's comments on his views of himself and his environment, his expressions of emotions, and problem areas. Guidance for intervention is related solely to improvement of communications but not for intervention into other pathology.

GUIDES FOR COMMUNICATION SKILLS I

Directions: Complete the Guide for Communication Skills I by selecting appropriate material from your first two recordings.

1. It is important that the client be able to receive and send stimuli as well as understand that which is received.
   a. Does the client have any physical difficulties in hearing, speaking, or understanding?

   b. Does the client have a language barrier resulting from the use of a foreign language or a regional dialect?

   c.   List any factors in the environment that may interfere with communi-
        cation.

   2.   Describe means available to you to alleviate difficulties you have observed
in the preceding areas.

   3.   Evaluate your intervention. Include the apparent reasons for the result.

   4.   If your intervention was not successful, suggest an alternate means. State
your reasons for thinking that your alternate plan may be successful.

5. Communication by the nurse must be specific and concise. Sentences should be short and direct.

    a. From your recording list the number of long sentences you used. Rephrase the sentences so that they contain the information you wished to give in a more direct manner.

    b. List the number of times you used vague terminology. List the terminology. Rephrase the vague terminology so that it is concise and concrete.

    c. Describe the instances in which you gave an incomplete description or explanation. Rephrase these examples so that they are complete, concise, concrete, and accurate.

d. How did you know your description or explanation was incomplete, inaccurate, or unclear?

e. Describe any reaction by your client that you think was related to your difficulties in presenting descriptions or explanations.

f. List the allegories, similes, metaphors, or abstract terminology you used. Rephrase them in concrete terms.

6. It is not always possible to understand the meaning the client is attempting to convey.

a. List any words or phrases used by the client that you did not understand.

b. Indicate your response to the communications you did not understand. Include the result of your response.

c. List examples of the use of loose associations by the client.

d. Describe your attempt to help the client explain the loose associations. Include the result of your intervention.

7. The client's communication reveals his understanding and interpretation of external stimuli reaching him. From your recording, try to see how the client views his world.
   a. What does the client say that indicates he is misinterpreting the communications of others?

b.   What does he say that indicates his understanding of other people?

c.   What does he say that indicates understanding of the nonhuman environment?

d.   What does he say that indicates he is misinterpreting the nonhuman environment?

e.   What are the reality factors in his misinterpretations?

8. The client's communications reveal his emotions.
    a. What does the client say that indicates the following emotions?
       (1) Anxiety

       (2) Depression

       (3) Suspicion

       (4) Hostility

       (5) Unreality

(6) Happiness

(7) Loneliness

(8) Apathy

(9) Optimism

9. The client's communication reveals his opinion of himself.
   a. How does the client describe himself?

b. How does the client describe his abilities?

c. What does the client say that indicates how he sees himself in relation to others?

d. Does he think he is important to anyone? If so, to whom?

e. How does the client describe his mental health?

    f.   What does the client say about his future role in his family and community?

GUIDE FOR COMMUNICATION SKILLS II

Directions: Complete the Guide for Communication Skills II by selecting material from any four recordings made during the working phase of the relationship and after completion of the Guide for Communication Skills I.

    1.   Describe areas of improvement in the client's ability to communicate accurately and completely. Include apparent reasons for the improvement.

    2.   Describe areas of improvement in your ability to communicate accurately and completely. Include apparent reasons for the improvement.

3. Cue words which alert the nurse to problem areas are described as cognitive and affective. Both quality and quantity are of importance. List and count the number of cognitive words or phrases used, the number of affective words or phrases used, and compare the ratio of cognitive to affective words in the four recordings. Count a phrase or theme as one word. Include relevant material only, in the discussion of the weather that follows:

Example: *"It's a nice day today. The weatherman is predicting thunderstorms tonight. I am terrified of storms."*

    a. The first two statements are cognitive data about the weather, and should be counted only once.

    b. The affective word "terrified" is the cue to the relevance of "weather" as a theme. It should be counted as one affective theme.

    c. Identify the ratio as 1:1.

Cognitive	Times Used	Affective	Times Used	Ratio
Weatherman predicted	1	Terrified	1	1:1

Recording I

Cognitive Words	Times Used	Affective Words	Times Used	
Total			Total	Ratio

Recording II

Cognitive Words	Times Used	Affective Words	Times Used	
	Total		Total	Ratio

Recording III

Cognitive Words	Times Used	Affective Words	Times Used	
	Total		Total	Ratio

Recording IV

Cognitive Words	Times Used	Affective Words	Times Used	
	Total		Total	Ratio

4. List any recurring themes or topics from the cognitive words selected.

5. List any recurring affective words.

6. State any conclusions you have reached from the above data concerning indications of problem areas in your client's life.

7. Select one incident from your recordings in which you received a cue through the use of an affective word by the client. Describe your response, your attempt at clarification and exploration of more details and the client's responses.

8. Evaluate your responses and the client's as to their effectiveness in providing a complete description. Suggest changes for future attempts at obtaining complete descriptions.

9. Describe the effect of the level of anxiety on the use of cognitive vs. affective words.

GUIDE FOR COMMUNICATION SKILLS III

Directions: Complete the Guide for Communications Skills III by selecting appropriate material from your recording made just previous to termination.

1. Describe permanent physical difficulties your client has in communicating verbally. Include means he uses to compensate for the handicap.

2. Describe your client's ability to convey meaning to you.

3. Describe your ability to convey meaning to your client.

4. Describe your means of determining what meanings the client assigns to your communication.

5. Describe improvement in communication that the client has made since the first recordings. Include the apparent reasons for the change.

6. Describe your areas of improvement in communication since the beginning of the nurse-client relationship.

7. Describe any changes in the ability of the client to express emotional concerns by using affective words. Suggest reasons for the change.

8. Describe any changes in the use of affective words that indicate increasing control of emotions such as changing the word "love" to "like," or a decrease in the use of affective words, or an increase in the use of cognitive words.

INSTRUCTOR'S COMMENTS

CHAPTER 4

Nonverbal Behavior

Nonverbal behavior is a direct form of communication which gives the nurse-practitioner many cues to thoughts and feelings that the client may not be able or may not wish to express verbally. Behavior may be overt or covert, direct or disguised. Therefore, in order to understand the meaning conveyed by nonverbal behavior, the nurse must observe carefully and then attempt to validate her observations and resulting interpretations. For example, the client may state that he is comfortable and at ease, yet a constant swinging of the foot and tapping of the fingers tell the nurse that the client is anxious. To validate her interpretation the nurse may comment to the client on her observations or may prefer postponing validation to a later time as her judgment dictates.

The manner in which the client presents himself to others gives a cue to emotion that may not be expressed. Posture, facial expression, and general appearance are commonly observed indications of emotion. Many times one aspect of nonverbal communication reinforces the others. The furrowed brow, the lines of the face pulled downward, or the lack of facial animation takes on added meaning when accompanied by stooped shoulders that appear to bear the burden of the world and by a general motor retardation. Add to this picture clothing that is dark and possibly in need of cleaning, a lack of jewelry and make-up, and hair and skin that need attention; the aura of despondency, sadness, and not-caring is vividly expressed without resorting to words. Contrast such an appearance with the person who is smiling and laughing, moving about quickly, and wearing a great deal of make-up and jewelry, and whose clothing, which although disheveled, is bright and gaudy.

The client's posture may express withdrawal from others. He may habitually sit alone in a corner or curl in a fetal position in a chair, on the floor, or covered by blankets in bed. When compelled to interact with others, he may avoid eye contact or sit or stand in such a way that he can exclude others from his presence as much as possible.

Many times posture gives the nurse her first clue that the client is hallucinating. She may observe him in a listening attitude or apparently looking at something or sniffing at something. Clues such as these need validation, however, before the nurse can hazard an interpretation.

Nonverbal behavior during the nurse-client interaction may give the nurse an indication of the client's reaction to the situation. Inability to approach the nurse, tardiness, leaving early, and silence may result from anxiety and conflict. Silence may also be used in an aggressive, withholding manner to make the nurse uncomfortable.

The client may present himself in a sexually provocative manner as a result of his misinterpretation of the nurse's attempts to establish a therapeutic relationship. The nonverbal behavior of the nurse may unconsciously cause or contribute to such a misinterpretation. Every action of the nurse may be interpreted by the client as being somehow related to him, so that if she wears a short skirt and uses a heavy perfume he may see this as designed to attract him. Sitting on the client's bed or bedside table may also be misinterpreted.

Intrusion of the personal space that the client considers his own may be indicated by a general uneasiness or an actual physical moving away. Each individual has his own idea of the personal space with which he is comfortable. The nurse can test her own personal space by requesting others to stand close to her, behind her, at a great distance, or at a "comfortable" distance. The "comfortable" distance indicates the boundaries of her own personal space. Physical closeness is anxiety-producing to many clients, as is physical distance, the one indicating intrusion, the other disapproval, disapprobation, or some other negative response. The nurse identifies the client's personal space only through experience and observation.

During the course of the nurse-client relationship, the client may identify closely with the nurse. Nonverbal indications of such identification may become apparent to the nurse as she observes the client imitating her gestures or otherwise assuming nonverbal behavior similar to her own.

Nonverbal behavior is not always readily interpreted. The nurse may think her client is sad but learn later that he was merely physically tired. Therefore, to avoid misinterpreting her observations, she will need to seek some validation of what she has observed and of the conclusions she has reached. Following validation, nursing intervention may occur in a realistic manner. Evaluation of the intervention increases the value of the experience by giving the nurse information that she may use in other experiences.

The following chart gives an example of observation, interpretation, validation, intervention, and evaluation of nonverbal behavior.

Directions: From your observations, select an example of nonverbal behavior. Describe it on the form provided below.

OBSERVATION OF BEHAVIOR

Nonverbal Behavior	Interpretations of Behavior	Apparent Reasons for Behavior	Validation by Observer	Nursing Intervention	Result of Intervention	Evaluation of Intervention	Suggestion for Change
1. Pulling skin at neck 2. Licking lips 3. Sweating 4. Dilation of pupils of eyes 5. Tightening of facial and general musculature 6. Rapid breathing	1. Client is anxious	1. Meeting with nurse	1. Asked client if she were uncomfortable. Reply affirmative.	1. Asked client what made her uncomfortable.	1. Discussion concerning feelings about meeting people. 2. Anxiety appeared to lessen during discussion.	1. Client helped to understand and accept her anxiety.	1. None

Directions: From your observations, select an example of nonverbal behavior. Describe it on the form provided below.

OBSERVATION OF BEHAVIOR

Nonverbal Behavior	Interpretations of Behavior	Apparent Reasons for Behavior	Validation by Observer	Nursing Intervention	Result of Intervention	Evaluation of Intervention	Suggestion for Change

GUIDE FOR OBSERVATION AND INTERPRETATION OF NONVERBAL BEHAVIOR

Part I

Select material from the orientation phase to complete the following items.

1. Describe your client's posture:
   a. Sitting

   b. Standing

   c. Walking

   d. When apparently unobserved

   e. When with you

2. Describe your client's facial expression
   a. When unobserved

   b. When greeting you

c. When leaving you

3. Describe your client's appearance in respect to
    a. Personal hygiene

    b. Clothing

    c. Use of cosmetics and jewelry

4. Explain any meaning that the client's posture, facial expression, and personal appearance may have. Describe your validation of the interpretation of the preceding.

5. Describe gestures your client uses. When does he use them? What is their effect?

6. Describe any mannerisms your client displays. When does he use them? Do they become exaggerated or increase for any reason? Why?

7. Describe your client's nonverbal behavior during nurse-client interactions.
    a. Physical approach to the meetings: Is he on time? Does he hesitate? Is he late?

    b. Seating arrangements: Does he face you? Does he face away from you? Does he sit beside you? Does he sit near you? Is he unable to sit? How does he sit? Who made the seating arrangements? How do they affect the nurse interaction?

    c. Professional relationship: Does any nonverbal behavior suggest that the client does not understand or is not maintaining the professional aspects of the relationship? Describe it and state a reason for its apparent cause.

d. Silence: When and how often is the client silent? Validate a reason for the silences. Describe his behavior during a silence. If your client is mute, how does he make his needs known? How effective is his method?

e. Describe any nonverbal indications of anxiety. Indicate possible causes of the anxiety, your validation of both the anxiety and its cause, and your subsequent interaction. Evaluate your intervention.

f. Does the client touch you? If so, when and for what apparent reason? How do you feel about the patient touching you?

g. Identify the boundaries of the client's personal space. How did you determine the boundary?

Just as the nonverbal behavior of the client communicates his feelings to you, so, too, does your nonverbal behavior give the client opportunity to assess your emotions. The nurse must make a decision when it will be helpful to allow the client to observe her emotional reactions and when it may be detrimental to him to do so. She must also decide how she will explain emotions inadvertently expressed. It is important, therefore, to become aware of unconscious mannerisms, such as twisting a strand of hair or picking at the skin, that may indicate anxiety. Posture that is strained, a voice that quavers or is strident, changes in respiration or complexion, facial expressions, swinging or tapping of the feet, and twisting the hands are all indicative of emotion which the client may interpret realistically or unrealistically.

8. Describe your own nonverbal behavior during the nurse-client interactions.

a. Your posture

b. Your facial expressions

c. Your use of gestures and mannerisms

d. Any behavior that may have contributed positively or adversely to the professional nature of the interaction

e.   Your behavior during a silence

f.   Any nonverbal behavior that is indicative of anxiety.

g.   Your touching the client. (Include your reasons for so doing and the client's reaction.)

h.   Describe the boundaries of your personal space.

i.   Describe your behavior when you are under stress.

j.   Ask a friend to describe your behavior when you are under stress.

k. How do you attempt to control your behavior so that you will not give indications that you are under stress? How successful are your attempts at concealment?

l. How will you attempt to control any display of emotion when you are with your client?

m. When will you wish to prevent your client from observing your emotions?

n. When will you wish to allow your client to become aware of your emotions?

Part II

Select material from recordings of the working phase to complete the following items.

1. Describe any new mannerisms or gestures the client is using. Are they similar to any that you use?

2. Describe any change in the physical appearance of the client that is indicative of his identifying with you.

3. Describe any other nonverbal behavior that seems to indicate that the client is identifying with you.

4. Describe any changes in nonverbal behavior that have occurred since the first interaction took place. Include the appearance of new nonverbal behavior. State your reasons for the changes and validate your interpretation.

Part III

Select material from the terminal phase to complete the following items.

1. Describe any nonverbal behavior by your client that indicates an increase in anxiety. Include your validation of your observations, your intervention, and your evaluation of your intervention.

2. Describe any nonverbal behavior on your part that indicates increasing anxiety. Describe its effect on the nurse-client relationship. Validate your interpretation of the effect of your anxiety.

3. Describe any nonverbal behavior that occurs now but did not take place during the previous phases. State any apparent reasons for such occurrences and validate your interpretation.

4. Describe any cessation of nonverbal behavior that occurred during the previous phases. Why do you think this behavior stopped?

INSTRUCTOR'S COMMENTS

CHAPTER 5

Assessing the Milieu

The milieu is the environment in which an individual exists. It consists of both human and nonhuman elements, the interactions between these elements, and the effects of the interactions. Some milieus are quite simple, some complex. Some are easily observable, some are well hidden. Each of us functions in more than one milieu; from a very personal, unique, private milieu, to a family, neighborhood, work, city, national, and international milieu. Each milieu has an effect on the other and on those in the milieu.

In assessing the milieus of her client, the nurse is faced with some basic questions. What is her client's world like? How does he fit in it? How did he get there? How is he maintained there? What effect does his position have on him? What effect does he have on others? What are the cultural traditions of his particular milieus? These may change rapidly between milieus! For example, a home milieu is very different from a work milieu. What is his most personal world like?

Personal worlds are unique to the individual and, therefore, of great importance in understanding a client. A good example of a personal world is that described by the child, Esther in "Bleak House" by Charles Dickens. A lonely child, she vividly describes hurrying home from school to her bedroom to talk over the day's troubles with her doll. Children frequently display the development of a private milieu as they seclude themselves under tables or beds or build tree houses or find a favorite spot in which to be alone.

Understanding the client involves understanding the various milieus and how elements in the milieus affect the client. Developing and implementing a care plan require that the nurse understand not only these effects but also how her client affects the milieus. She needs to be aware that when change occurs in the client, that change will affect the milieu. Many times a milieu is stabilized by maintaining a client in a state of illness. Therefore, bringing about adaptive behavior in the client will cause instability in the milieus. Change will be resisted by those to whose advantage it is to keep the client ill. For example, a sixty-five year old mother, in order to feel needed, necessary, and therefore, "well," maintained her forty year old son in a state of dependency. She provided total care for all of his needs, even to the extent of bathing him and washing his hair. In effect she was keeping him at the level of a two year old child. Any attempt by the son (diagnosed as chronic schizophrenic) to manage any self-care was viewed with alarm and actively discouraged. Intervention by a visiting nurse who suggested that the son might benefit from walking to the corner store, unaccompanied by his mother, resulted in the expulsion of the nurse.

In another instance, sudden improvement in the condition of a mentally ill wife resulted in just as sudden an appearance of severe mental illness in the husband.

The nurse, therefore, must assess what in the milieu affects the client, what effect the client is having in his milieus, and what may possibly happen if either the client or the milieu changes.

Beginning the assessment, the nurse may list the major milieus in which the client exists. For most people this would include a personal milieu, the home, a place of employment, and recreational milieus. It may be well to account for the amount of time spent in each area, but in so doing one must question whether one hour in hell is equivalent to eight hours in heaven.

It is apparent that the meaning the milieu has for the client is probably its most important aspect. However, for the sake of academic necessity, the usual impossible dichotomy between physical and mental aspects will be attempted.

THE PHYSICAL MILIEU

Major components of the physical milieu are those related to safety, comfort, and the provision of life-maintaining needs.

Safety factors are comparatively standardized. Obviously the presence of rats, vermin, dirt, broken stairs, faulty heating and plumbing equipment, rubbish, and garbage are not conducive to a safe milieu. Of particular concern to the very young or the elderly is danger from accidents, fire; or violence. Living for many years in such an environment may dull its impact on the client but, like knowledge of the horror of the hydrogen bomb, awareness is present and is a factor to be considered.

Life-maintaining needs are those basic elements without which life cannot exist. They differ from comfort needs, which will be discussed later, in that they represent minimal requirements. Life-maintaining needs represent existence, comfort needs represent the quality of that existence. Many people question the value of existence without quality, but no one can question the fact that without existence there can be no quality. Oxygen, water, food, shelter, and rest must be available to sustain life. In this country, lack of food is the first of the life-sustaining needs that the nurse must check. Occasionally water and shelter are not available, but, in general, malnutrition is more likely to be encountered.

Physical comfort in the milieu not only is more difficult to assess because it is related to the uniqueness of the individual, but also because it is closely related to psychological comfort. One is physically uncomfortable even in the most plush milieu if one is psychologically uncomfortable.

Physical comfort is based in part on the presence of items which help fulfill life's needs. The degree of accessibility to these items indicates a comfort measure. Water is a basic need. If one can turn on a faucet and obtain an adequate water supply rather than being obliged to walk to a well and draw water by bucket, that is a comfort need. A third floor apartment may limit the amount of exercise possible for an eighty year old client but she may find the 84 degree temperature in summer very comfortable. The reverse would be true of the adolescent.

Once the nurse has assessed comfort measures related to basic needs, she can enlarge her horizon to include items which add to the amenities of life. The presence of comfortable furniture and household items in sufficient amounts and in reasonable repair contribute to physical comfort. Luxury items such as automatic dishwashers, automatic clothes washers and dryers, self-cleaning ovens, color TV's, electric mixers, and blenders not only contribute to comfort but also help indicate the economic level of the client.

Once basic physical needs are assessed, the nurse begins to identify factors in the milieu which give cues to the client's personality. Care must be taken to realize that the economic level of the client will affect some of the measures he takes to arrange his milieu in his own inimitable fashion. For example, the client may not have photographs of his family in view because he cannot afford them. He may have no pictures or ornaments of any kind for the same reason. However, he also may have no photography, pictures, or ornaments because he will not spend money on "foolishness" or he cannot stand "clutter." Realizing thay many factors are involved in providing a milieu, the nurse does not make any immediate assumptions about what she observes or does not observe.

A first impression is important because eventually the nurse may become so accustomed to the milieu that she loses her awareness. Using four, maybe five, of her senses the nurse records her first impression as she observes it but without making any conclusions. When she first enters the client's home, what does she see? What does she smell? What does she hear? What do objects that she touches feel like? If she accepts a cup of coffee, how does it taste?

Once a general impression is gained, the nurse observes more closely. She looks for cues that tell her about her client in an intimate manner. Therefore, she tries to observe items which appear to be important to him. A particular area of the home may be set aside for specific occasions. For example, a living room may be reserved for formal guests, the kitchen for friends, and a basement room for adolescents. On the other hand, maybe there are no such arrangements and one sits wherever one happens to be. The nurse may be given a "tour" in which various objects are pointed out. What seems to be important on this tour? "This is the vase great-grandmother brought from the old country" or "This is the doggie bank we won at Coney Island." Instead of a tour, various family members may be introduced. "This is Johnnie. He's in the third grade and is getting all A's. This one is Harold. He's impossible. He's in the seventh grade, doesn't mind, and has been suspended twice."

The nurse assesses the value the client seems to place on inanimate objects. Which seems to be of greater importance? May Mary Anne coming home from school have a peanut butter sandwich or must she eat a cookie instead to avoid making a mess with the peanut butter? What happens to the pictures the first grader brings home? Are they prominently displayed or are they shoved out of sight? What about the family dog? Is he treated kindly or is he abused? Does he take the place of a child? Does housework take precedence over child care? For example, what happens when a parent is involved in a necessary household task and a child interrupts seeking attention?

Some interesting observations can be made about inanimate objects. What is their value to the client? Is it their color, their form, an idea they represent? Are pictures of people or are they of objects or landscapes? What colors seem to predominate? Are they of the client's choosing?

The nurse's assessment of physical comfort needs narrows still more as she attempts to identify a specific niche that is the client's. Perhaps he does not have one. Perhaps nothing in the milieu seems to be his and his alone. Perhaps his niche consists of a specific chair or room. Why is this his area? What is its value? What does he see or hear from it? Where is it? Does it isolate him or protect him from others or is he included in a family grouping?

Closely related to the comfort of having a personal space is having a personal time. Most people have a certain time which they can call their own to use for their own purposes. For many housewives this personal time occurs as the last child leaves on the school bus and the husband leaves for work. She can then sit down for five minutes before resuming the work of the day. For others, the personal time consists of "watching the evening news on TV" For still others, it occurs as a bedtime ritual. Most individuals part with this personal time grudgingly and with irritation. Encroachment by others may be met with a seemingly disproportionate display of anger and annoyance over what appears to be a trivial circumstance. After all, if the evening news is missed, the world will not really fall apart. The violence of the response indicates to the observer the serious meaning to the client of his personal comfort time. If no such personal time can be demonstrated, an indication of serious pathology exists.

It may be a long while before the nurse can identify comfort measures in the client's most intimate, personal milieu, the one which consists of that which the client truly cherishes.

THE PSYCHOLOGICAL MILIEU

As can be seen from the foregoing, much that is psychological crept into the discussion of the physical environment. In the beginning of the relationship, the nurse more readily observes the physical milieu because it is tangible. As the relationship progresses, however, she intensifies her assessment of they psychological milieu. Her assessment can be divided roughly into two major areas, first, the meanings attached to the physical milieu, and second, the interplay of personal relationships and their meanings. In making her physical assessment, the nurse observes. In making a psychological assessment, the nurse analyzes.

Many items bear meaning one would expect. For example, photographs of relatives, friends, or a favorite vacation spot are prized because of the memories involved. A simple gift from a cherished friend has meaning, not because of its monetary worth, but as an indication of a close relationship. Lack of meaning for items which are usually cherished may be significant and should be noted, although with some caution. There are people who find photographs unappealing yet sustain intense, warm relationships. Lack of any cherished items indicates an impoverished milieu and is quite significant, unless circumstances are such that the client is allowed no personal possessions. When a client finds nothing to be of value, he may also find life meaningless and not worth sustaining.

It may become apparent that some objects bear meanings for the client that are quite unique and appear inappropriate to the object. This may be a cue that there are delusional or phantasied ideas attached to the object. For example, a client caring for a kitten in an extremely solicitous manner consulted her as to how, when, and where she wanted her milk; whether it was permissible for the client to leave the apartment; how much money should be spent; and so on. Eventually, the client explained that the kitten was really the Virgin Mary. Cues such as these may occur in less extreme form and do give interesting side lights into the behavior of very normal people. A brother "borrowed" his sister's Girl Scout knife at the age of ten. Now, in his forties, while he jokes about the knife, he still keeps it! Careful observation over a period of time will reveal values of this kind and will provide fruitful avenues for the nurse to explore. The nurse then needs to assess what objects the client values and why he values them.

The most cogent factor in the milieu is the interplay of actions and reactions between individuals. It is not the purpose of this workbook to elaborate extensively on the family or group dynamics and their related therapies. The major concern here is with one individual, one client. However, no one lives in a vacuum and, therefore, it is necessary to observe interactions between those in a specific milieu. Such observations will affect the nursing care plan for the individual since it will suggest strengths and weaknesses in the milieu which must be accounted for if the nursing care plan is to succeed.

On entering a milieu, the nurse must be aware that her presence changes it. She may find family members very polite and friendly both to her and to each other. She may find also that the family uses her as a captive audience to describe the failings of each other. She may be treated as an intruder and discover the family will close ranks so that they present a solid front against her. In any event, her major purpose is to maintain a relationship with her client. Therefore, her objective is to determine principally how her client interacts with others, how others interact with him, and the results of these interactions.

Earlier in the chapter, in assessing the physical milieu, the nurse observed whether the client had a personal niche and where it was in relation to others. She then assesses the meaning of the location of the niche or even the lack of a personal area. Perhaps the assessment most familiar to a student is to remember seating arrangements at meal time in her own home. Who sat where and what happened if someone sat in the "wrong" place? How do places get assigned? What changes them? What happens when change does occur? Think back to other milieus such as the school room. The nurse can usually identify her own pattern of selecting a place and, with a little concentration, figure out why she chooses as she does.

The status of the client within the milieu can also be identified by listening to statements made by others. How he is addressed can be a cue. Nicknames have a tendency to stick from childhood to old age, but some of them can be belittling. For example, "Tony" for Anthony is a friendly, warm, accepting diminutive but "Tony Baby" addressed to a forty year old man may indicate that he has less than adult status.

The use of a pronoun rather than a proper name gives the appearance of non-identity as does discussing the client's condition in his presence, as though he were not there. Such behavior is not confined to custodial, outmoded "asylums". The following conversation was reported by a student nurse after her first visit to the home of a client. She was met by the client's sister who "introduced" her to the client and then proceeded at length to catalogue a series of problems while the client listened.

> "Hi! This is her. I don't know what you think you can do with her. She's been like this for five years now. She always looks like a slob. Look at her! She's got orange juice and eggs all over her face but she doesn't care. She doesn't care about anything. She just sits in that chair all day. We took the rockers off it because she used to rock all day and nearly drove me crazy. She never helps me. I got all this housework and she never even wipes the dishes. You talk to her and she doesn't hear you. You can't do nothing with her. I don't know why you want to try but I guess you'll have to find out the hard way. What are you going to do with her anyway?"

From this beginning introduction, the nurse identified that the client had a specific place, her chair, that she was viewed as a "her" rather than a person, that she was not pleasant to look at, that she made no tangible contribution to the physical care of the milieu, that she was considered hopeless, and that she made no response to the status in which she was placed by the sister. Removing the rockers from the chair and cataloguing her "vices" openly and to a stranger indicate both hostility and frustration on the part of the sister. The lack of response by the client presented the nurse with a cue which could be explored once the relationship was established.

When all the family members are present, the nurse attempts to observe who is in control of the situation. Control can switch from one person to another, be vested in one person only, or be exercised by no one, with a chaotic situation resulting. At this point, the nurse is concerned with power or lack of it so that she may use it to help the client. If she were doing family therapy, her interest might be centered in intervening in a maladaptive power structure, but in this instance, although she may bring about some changes, her chief focus is the single client. As stated earlier, the client cannot be treated as an isolated figure. Others in the milieu must be considered. The nurse will necessarily become involved to some degree, if only in explaining what she is doing and in seeking family assistance. However, her major intervention is with her client. In family therapy the focus is on the entire family unit. In a one-to-one relationship the focus is on the client.

The nurse observes the power structure within the family because it tells her whether the milieu is autocratic, democratic, laissez-faire, or chaotic. Her care plan will be materially affected by this observation. Care must be taken not to base a decision on the client's report or on any other family member's report. Many clients will report thay they are being totally controlled by others, while in actual fact the client may be exercising a great deal of power either actively or passively.

Emotional tone of the milieu is another difficult factor which must be assessed. Extremes of hate, anxiety, apathy, or concern are easily noted but lesser emotional states may be masked and much more difficult to discern. The nurse must also be aware of her own emotional state and not project it to the milieu she is observing. A nurse anxious over her first meeting with a client may identify that anxiety as a "tense milieu" without realizing that the tension is more hers than the client's. The physical assessment of the milieu can supply some clues to a prevailing emotional tone. A house in which nothing is ever dirty, dusty, or out of place, in which everything is done exactly on schedule is a tense, anxious household. In visiting a children's ward, the author noted just such a situation. All the children were dry, very clean, seated quietly in cribs, and numbers of brightly colored toys were tastefully arranged totally out of reach of the children. The little sad faces are impossible to forget.

In contrast is the chaotic household where nothing belongs anywhere even if anywhere can be found. In just such a household, one of the children had not gone to school because he could not find his shoes. It was suggested to the mother that a second youngster, age four, could use some soap and water. Her reply, as she continued to drink a cup of instant coffee, was "Why? He'll only get dirty again." A dead dog in the kitchen was finally removed a week later—removed to the cellar anyway!

In facing either milieu, the nurse may well feel both helpless and hopeless. Sometimes, however, it is easier to work in such extremes because they are so tangible and change can actually be observed. The milieu which is the most difficult is that in which, superficially, there appears to be no problem. Eventually, the nurse may be cued by a carefully casual remark by the client that will lead to the discovery of underlying anxiety, tension, or other disturbance. Passive aggression, manipulation, and neurotic behavior can be hidden so that all appears calm and pleasant. Here again, a physical cue may be the first indication the nurse has.

For example, a forty year old woman with many psychosomatic problems lived with her mother. The mother encouraged her daughter frequently to act independently although she did not force her in any way. Superficially, she was a charming, kind mother interested in trying to help her daughter in any way she could. The cue that the nurse gained to the mother's means of maintaining her daughter's dependency appeared when she noticed that all of the daughter's clothing was beautifully handmade in a style twenty years out of date. Even the stitching was done by hand, not by machine. In essence, what she was saying was "Look what a good mother I am. You cannot leave me." Obviously, the clothing was only a small indication but it gave the nurse a place to start investigating. She eventually became aware of a milieu in which the status of the daughter was revealed as a helpless, but "loved", child totally unattractive to her peers, and totally managed by her charming mother, a pleasant enough existence provided you have no desires or ideas of your own.

In family therapy, one is concerned with who relates to whom and how. In individual therapy, however, the concern is chiefly with how others relate to the client, how the client relates to others, and the overall atmosphere in which the client exists.

Most of the emphasis has been placed on the family milieu, but the same principles apply to other areas which the client frequents. The same observations relating to both the physical and psychological milieus apply. For example, a client recently discharged from a large state mental institution visited a nearby doughnut and coffee shop and told the nurse that she would never go again because "everyone stared at her and she had to wait twenty minutes for coffee despite the fact that the waitress was not busy." It is simple enough to dismiss this statement as being a distortion of reality by a client unaccustomed to being so independent. However, the nurse coaxed her into a return trip accompanying her to help "remove the distortion." The nurse noted that people on the street did indeed stare at her and the situation in the doughnut shop was precisely as the client reported it. The community had assigned the client the status of "crazy and dangerous." Similar problems may occur in a work situation.

Recreational milieus need special mention since many clients tend to gravitate toward areas where other individuals who have been mentally ill may be found. Drop In centers for discharged patients, social clubs, and informal groups of those who have been mentally ill serve a very useful purpose. However, many clients need to be encouraged to participate in recreational social activities such as church groups, the Y's, and other organizations in which the role of "mental patient" plays no part.

It appears almost inevitable that the client who has been mentally ill or has an emotional problem of some kind is going to have to face discrimination or disparaging remarks from someone. There are those in the community who still talk about "the loonies," "the nuts," and "crazy people", who think that to be mentally ill is to be dangerous, or is a stigma resulting from sin and weakness. This a part of the milieu and nurse and client must deal with it.

GUIDE TO ASSESSING THE MILIEU

General Observations

1. List the major milieus in which your client appears and indicate the approximate amount of time spent in each.

2.   State the milieu in which the client states he is most comfortable. Include his reasons for declaring it comfortable and the amount of time he spends in it.

3.   Compare your observations of the above milieu with the client's statements about it in respect to:

Client's Description	Your Observation
a. Meeting basic physical needs.	a.
b. Amount of interaction initiated by others with client. Include his response as he reports it.	b.
c. Quality of interaction initiated by others with client. Include his response as he reports it.	c.
d. General emotional tone.	d.

4. Describe what you have observed as positive in the milieu selected as comfortable.

5. Describe what you have observed as adverse in the milieu selected as comfortable.

6. Describe misconceptions, distortions of reality, or delusions the client has about the milieu and suggest any purpose these serve for the client.

7. Describe any interventions you attempted in the above situation and include the results. If you did not intervene, state your reasons for not doing so.

8. State the milieu in which the client states he is least comfortable. Include his reasons for his discomfort and the amount of time spent in it.

9. Compare the client's description of the milieu described as uncomfortable with your own observations.

Client's Description	Your Observation
a. Meeting basic physical needs.	a.
b. Meeting physical comfort needs.	b.
c. Status assigned client.	c.
d. Amount of interactions initiated by client with others. Include their response.	d.
e. Quality of interaction initiated by client with others.	e.

Client's Description   *Your Description*

f. Amount of interaction   f.
    initiated by others. In-
    clude client's responses.

g. Quality of interaction   g.
    initiated by others. In-
    clude client's responses.

h. General emotional tone.   h.

10. Describe what you observe as positive in the milieu.

11. Describe what you observe as negative in the milieu.

12.   Describe misconceptions, distortions of reality, or delusions the client has about the milieu and suggest any purpose these serve for the client.

13.   Describe any interventions you attempted in the above situation and include your results. If you did not intervene, state your reasons for not doing so.

14.   Identify any effect the comfortable milieu has on the less comfortable milieu and vice versa.

THE PERSONAL MILIEU

The personal milieu refers to that milieu which is uniquely the client's. Elements of this personal space may be transported back and forth between various milieus or may be kept as a closely guarded secret. In any event, the personal milieu is that which carries the most meaning for the client. The nurse may not become totally aware of this milieu for a long time, if ever.

1. From your observations of the milieu which the client describes as most comfortable, identify:

  a. Any physical space that appears to be considered solely the client's. Is this space respected and accepted by others?

  b. Any inanimate objects that the client appears to cherish. Include his reasons for valuing the objects, the reactions of others to these objects, and his response to any threat against these objects.

  c. Any animate objects other than humans that the client values. Describe his behavior with such objects and the responses of others to his behavior, and to the objects.

  d. Any intense relationships with humans in this milieu. Describe his behavior and their response.

e. Any specific time that the client describes as his own. Include his activities during this time and the reaction of others to his personal time. What happens if his time is interrupted?

f. Approximately how much time during the day is the client involved solely in his personal milieu?

2. In the milieu which the client has indicated as being uncomfortable, describe any evidence you observe of his including a personal milieu. (Examples may be family pictures on a desk, special wearing apparel, favorite tools, trophies, special space.) Include the responses of others to his personal milieu. What happens if he loses some of his personal milieu?

3. In the milieu which the client describes as uncomfortable, how much time can he find to remove himself temporarily from its stress? How does he do this, how effective is his avoidance, and what are the responses of others?

4. If you cannot observe any personal milieu in which your client functions, how do you account for this apparent lack?

5. Identify any unrealistic factors in any of the client's personal milieus. Indicate the apparent purpose of unreality factors and the responses of others.

6. What does the client gain from his personal milieu?

7. Describe any adverse effects of the client's maintenance of his personal milieu in relation to:
   a. Time

   b. Space

   c. Inanimate objects

   d. Nonhuman animate objects

   e. Relationships with other humans

8. Describe the chief values to the client of his personal milieu.

9. Identify strengths in the personal milieu.

10. Identify weaknesses in the personal milieu.

11. Milieus common to most individuals are the home, place of work, and a recreational-social milieu. Does the client function in all of these milieus? Identify any that are missing in your client's life and suggest any reasons for the lack.

INSTRUCTOR'S COMMENTS

CHAPTER 6

Trust

The establishment of a basis for trust is essential in the formation of a therapeutic relationship between the nurse and her client. Trust in the nurse will help the client to learn from her. Trust in the client will help the nurse to accept him as a unique and valuable individual. In the nurse-client relationship, trust is a mutual expectation of the essential reliability of each member. The nurse may bring with her a general sense of trust that is founded on her past experience that others are friendly and trustworthy. The client, however, frequently brings a sense of mistrust, validly or invalidly based on his experience that others are hostile and not to be trusted. When in the past he accepted a relationship of trust, too often he found, or thought he found, that the trust was broken. With each succeeding betrayal, the ability to trust became weaker and the client became more conscious of elements in a relationship with another that indicated a lack of integrity. Minor disturbances in a relationship increasingly assumed major proportions as the client actively looked for indications of unreliability. Distortion of perception gave the client the final proof he sought, that the world is indeed hostile and not to be trusted.

There are many subtle variables, originating in the client's unique past and unknown to the nurse, which arouse mistrust within him. A great many clients, particularly those who are mentally ill, have suffered from a series of experiences, particularly in the first years of life, that have caused them to think that others are not reliable. When significant people consistently failed to meet the demands or needs of the client as an infant, he interpreted the world in general as being hostile, indifferent, unfriendly, and painful. However, some of his needs must have been met on some occasions or the infant would have died. Therefore, as an infant, he learned that sometimes he would be cared for, but he was unable to tell when "sometime" would be or why it occurred. Unable to determine when or why his needs would be met, he concluded that he was not able to depend on others to meet his needs. In other words, he learned a basic mistrust of other people, of his own ability to procure help, and of his environment in general.

As the client grew from infancy to childhood and acquired the ability to communicate verbally, he may actively have sought answers to his problem. When answers that were given were not true or were given in such a way that their meaning was obscured, the feeling of mistrust was reinforced. Nonverbal behavior that conflicted with verbal communications added to the confusion and mistrust that he experienced as a child. Promises that may have been made to the child were subsequently broken, with or without adequate explanations.

As a child it is possible that he might have heard his faults and misdemeanors openly discussed before others, or he may have been allowed to exhibit behavior in public which was later condemned, leaving him to believe that he was unable to depend on those who were caring for him to protect him from censure and ridicule. He may have shared information that he considered confidential with significant people to find that again his trust was betrayed as his secrets were revealed indiscriminately.

The tenuous trust he may have been able to develop would have been badly shaken if the person who cared for him left without explaining the absence or without leaving some familiar person as a substitute. He saw the absence as absolute rejection or abandonment. Temporary or short absences, as well as long absences can cause the feeling of loss or abandonment, particularly since the child has already learned that other significant people are unreliable and cannot be trusted to provide care.

In all interpersonal relationships, there are many common factors that will encourage trust. Scrupulous attention must be paid to these details when the nurse is attempting to establish a therapeutic relationship with a mentally ill client, particularly since he is not only aware of minor transgressions but is actively looking for and expecting them to occur. For this reason an explicit contract is made with the client so that he will have some predictable events in which he may trust. Usually the terms of the contract include specific facts related to the date, time, and place of meetings, the duration of each meeting, the purpose of the meetings, the roles of both client and nurse, the use of information acquired, the use and control of recordings, and the termination date. Arrangements are also made to notify the client in case of unavoidable delay or absence of the nurse, so that even if the communication lines are broken, the client has the assurance that the nurse will attempt to notify him.

Once the terms of the contract are clear, the client can begin to learn and then trust that the nurse will arrive at a designated area on time as she promised. He may observe that the nurse, in turn, has trust in him that he will maintain the contract and will come to the meeting place on time. This she shows by not looking for the client when he fails to appear, provided she knows that he is oriented to time, place, and the terms of the contract and is capable of maintaining the agreement.

Honesty concerning all factors of the nurse-client relationship helps form a beginning basis for trust. The mechanics of the relationship, such as time and place of meeting, are clearly stated and maintained as previously described. The nurse also states that a specified time has been set aside for the exclusive use of the client. Therefore, she allows nothing short of national disaster to interfere with the meeting, whether or not the client maintains the contract. This means not only that she arrives on time at a previously designated area, but that she remains there for the length of time already set aside for the specific use of her client. If her client does not join her, she may or may not seek him out to remind him of the meeting, depending on individual circumstances. However, she continues to keep the specified time free so that she is available to the client and the client knows she is accessible. When other clients approach her, she must tactfully explain that her time is reserved for the sole use of her client. Sitting quietly and waiting for a client who may not appear is one of the more difficult and frustrating tasks of the novice student. Making home visit after visit only to find the client is away, is also most discouraging.

The nurse states that the purpose of the meetings is for the sole use of the client. To introduce irrelevant material such as a lengthy discussion of the weather or of a party attended by the nurse is to deny the contract. Likewise, it is a violation to ask direct questions about the client's problems no matter how relevant the nurse may think such information to be. If she has stated that the purpose of the meetings is for the client to talk about whatever he wishes, then she must abide by the agreement and wait until the client introduces whatever he thinks is important. The student is very likely to encounter long and painful silences, which she may be tempted to break solely to relieve her own discomfort. When she does so, her comments or questions may not reflect subject matter that is of concern to the client at that moment because only he can make such a judgment. The student may think that a direct question will help the client "get started," and it may produce something of note, but it does violate the contract and it may not refer to the problem that is disturbing the client at that moment. When the nurse's judgment tells her that a silence is causing anxiety that is too painful and intolerable, or that the client is using the silence in a negative manner, such as to withdraw, she may break the silence by commenting on the silence itself without damaging trust. Her comment that the silence makes her uncomfortable may relieve some of the tension. It may also show the client that the nurse is being honest with him by her admission of her own discomfort. He also may gain trust by observing that the nurse has recognized his anxiety and is attempting to alleviate it.

He will gain further trust in the nurse when he learns that if he is unable to control his behavior, the nurse will help him set limits rather than reject him or allow him to expose himself to the censure of others. With help, he can learn to express his emotions, express them constructively, and eventually trust himself to cope with the tremendous emotional storms that beset him. When the client threatens to break windows, the nurse may suggest that he pound his pillow as a substitute. Possibly she may seek help from other personnel to physically prevent the client from carrying out his threat. If he is successful in carrying out his threat, the nurse may accept his behavior as being a destructive means of relieving his hostility, describe it as such to him, and suggest alternate means for relieving hostility. Although disapproval of the client's behavior may be expressed, the continuation of the nurse-client relationship may prove to him that he is acceptable even if his behavior is not. He may be led to feel that the nurse has trust in his ability to eventually react to stress in a neutral or constructive manner rather than a destructive way.

Many times a client questions the efficacy of the help being offered him or the professional ability of personnel administering care. The nurse's views may coincide with those of the client, but her professional obligations will not allow her to express them if they happen to be derogatory. Furthermore, it would hardly seem therapeutic to damage the client's sense of security by intimating that his care is inadequate. The nurse may use any questions the client may have to help clarify his attitudes toward others, particularly those in authority. In so doing, she may expose misconceptions that the client has acquired. She may also have to explain her professional role if she may not answer the client's question. The client can then see that the nurse will help to untangle his misconceptions, will perhaps help correct his attitudes toward others, and finally may be trusted to maintain her professional role in her relations with others.

To establish a basis for trust is a time-consuming, vital requirement. To maintain trust is a never-ending task which is tested and proved daily. The goal of the nurse is to establish a basis for trust so that the client may accept her as a person who is helping him and on whom he can rely.

The following guide contains a series of items related to the establishment and maintenance of trust. As stated previously, the task of building trust is a continuous one. Therefore, it is not possible to isolate selected recordings, such as the first five or the last three, to complete the guide. It is suggested that the student familiarize herself with the various items and then complete the guide as different experiences related to the building of trust occur in the relationship.

GUIDE FOR ESTABLISHMENT OF TRUST

Review the terms of your contract with the client, particularly in relation to time and place of meeting, length of meeting, content of interviews, and use and confidentiality of data.

Mechanics of the Relationship

1. What arrangements have you made to inform the client if you are going to be unavoidably late or absent from the interview?

What evidence do you have that your arrangements will be effective?

What will you personally say to the client if you are late or absent?

2.   List the times you have been late or absent and the reasons for your absence.

Was the client informed in advance of your intention to be late or absent? What was his response when he received the information?

What was the client's response to your explanation?

3. List the times the client has been late or absent for the interview.

Were you given the information that he would be late? By whom? What did you do or say? How did you feel?

Describe the client's explanation for his absence.

If the client did not offer an explanation for his absence, what did you say or do? State your reasons for your choice of action.

If the client continues to be late or absent, what will you say or do? State your reasons for your choice of action.

4. What length of time did you specify that each interview would last?

Have you shortened or lengthened their duration? If so, why did you do so?

What explanation did you give the client? What was his response to the change in time and to your explanation?

Has the client shortened or lengthened the interviews? By how much?

What reasons did the client give for the change in duration?

What was your response to the change and to the client's explanation? State your reasons for your response.

If the client offered no explanation for the change, what will you do? Why?

The interview time is for the exclusive use of your client. What will you do if another person attempts to involve you or your client in another activity?

What will you do if hospital or clinic personnel or family interrupt the interview?

5. Has the place of meeting been changed? If so, by whom was the change made and for what reasons? What was the result of the change?

6. Describe briefly the content of the interviews directly related to the client and his problems.

Describe the content not related to the client and his problems.

How often did you introduce irrelevant material into the interviews? Why did you do so?

How did you explain the introduction of irrelevant material to the client? What was his response?

How often did the client introduce irrelevant material? What was the apparent reason for the use of irrelevancies? What was the stated reason for the use of irrelevancies?

How will you keep the content of the interviews to your stated purpose?

How can you use the introduction of irrelevant material during the interviews to increase the client's trust in you?

Has the client asked to see recordings of the interviews? If so, what has been his response to reading them?

What did you tell the client about safeguarding the recordings so that the material in them remains confidential?

What has the client said that indicates he feels the recordings are safe or not safe from the intrusion of others?

Dynamics of Trust

1. Describe what you interpret as evidence that the client is able to trust you.

2. Describe your trust in the client in relation to his maintaining the terms of your contract.

3. Describe any change in the quality of the client's communications that may indicate a beginning of trust.

Describe any change in nonverbal behavior that you interpret as evidence that the client is able to trust you.

Describe any changes in your verbal communications that you feel are a result of increased trust of your client.

Describe any changes in your nonverbal communications that you feel are a result of increased trust of your client.

4. Describe any time when you told the client you would perform a service for him or carry out some activity and then were unable to do so.

What was the client's response?

What was your explanation and his response to your explanation?

What reason did the client give for not performing the service himself or asking help of people other than you?

5. Describe any attempt the client has made to determine your intention of maintaining the contract between you.

Describe any attempt the client has made to discourage you or frighten you so that you will break the contract.

Are you afraid of your client? If so, of what are you afraid? What indications has the client given to cause your fear?

What will you do about controlling your fear?

Is the client aware of your fear? How do you know that he is aware of your fear?

Have you made any attempt to break the contract between you and your client? If so, why?

Has the client given any indication that he thinks you would like to break the contract? How did you intervene to relieve his doubts if they were unfounded? What were the results of your intervention?

If you did wish to break the contract or gave such indications, how did you explain your desire to the client?

What was his response?

Describe any indications that the client is afraid of you.

Describe any reasons the client has given for his fear.

How have you helped the client control his fear?

What other means are available to help the client control his fear?

What indications do you have that the client trusts his own ability to control his fear?

6.   On the following pages, list questions that the client has asked about himself or his problem that if honestly answered may cause him to be anxious or hurt. List your answers with the questions and your reasons for so answering. Examples of such questions are:

> "Am I crazy?"
> "Will I ever get out of here?"
> "Am I like those crazy patients?"
> "Will I get well?"

Question

Answer

Reason for Answer

Question	Answer	Reason for Answer

What were the client's responses? Evaluate your answers and the client's responses in relation to the establishment or maintenance of trust between you.

7. On the following pages, list questions that the client has asked about his environment and the people in it, which if honestly answered may cause the client to lose trust in others or to doubt their value. List your answers and state your reasons for so answering. Examples of such questions are:

"How can I get better in this dirty hole?"
"How can I get better when the doctor only sees
    me for a few minutes each week?"
"Why should I talk to a student? How can you
    help me if you are just learning?"
"The doctor doesn't understand. He's a foreigner."
"How can he help me when he doesn't know what
    I'm talking about?"
"He is sicker than I am. How can he help?"
"Welfare Dept. said they would help me. Why
    haven't they?"

Question	Answer	Reason for Answer

Question

Answer

Reason for Answer

What were the client's responses? Evaluate your answers and the client's response in relation to establishing or maintaining trust in you and in other people.

8. Describe an experience in which the client exhibited socially unacceptable behavior in your presence.

Describe your intervention or lack of intervention, state the reasons for your behavior, and describe the client's response to intervention.

9. To whom or where does your client go when he needs help? Describe his methods of obtaining help from others. Include the kind of help he expects and the results of his seeking.

10. With what kinds of problems does the client seek help? With what problems does he need help but does not seek it? What causes him to seek or not seek help?

11. Evaluate your intervention in the experiences described under items 8, 9, and 10 in relation to the establishment of trust between you, your client and other people in his environment.

INSTRUCTOR'S COMMENTS

CHAPTER 7

Acceptance

Acceptance of another is a means of expressing belief in the intrinsic worth of that person. The worth is seen despite behavior that appears to be unacceptable. Acceptance by the nurse does not imply permissiveness but rather indicates that she sees the worth in her client, while realizing that much unacceptable behavior is a manifestation of illness or of poorly developed skill in relating to others. Belief in the worth of the individual client leads the nurse to set limits on behavior so that his worth may develop as he is set free from maladaptive behavior.

Acceptance of another person is marked by the realization that differences in values occur not only between various cultures but even within the confines of a tightly knit family unit. Recognition of these differences and the right of the individual to maintain them curtails the tendency to dole out advice or to inflict one's own standards and values on another. The expression "If I were you, I would . . ." becomes meaningless in a therapeutic setting. I am not someone else nor can I become someone else. Therefore, just as I am unable to accept totally the values of another, so he is unable to accept mine.

Many clients with emotional problems have experienced rejection rather than acceptance. Therefore, they have difficulty not only in seeing themselves as acceptable but in accepting others. As a result, they may test the nurse to determine whether she will continue to maintain the contract she has established. Breaking the contract not only betrays trust but also reinforces the client's belief that he is not an acceptable person.

GUIDE FOR ACCEPTANCE

Directions: Complete the following items from your experiences with your client or with others as indicated by the questions. Include dates and verbatim recordings where possible.

1. Why did you select the client you did with whom to establish a nurse-client relationship?

2. Describe characteristics of your client of which you approve.

3. Describe characteristics of your client which you find pleasing.

4. Describe characteristics of your client of which you disapprove.

5. Describe characteristics of your client which you dislike or find annoying.

6. Describe characteristics of your client that are usually considered socially unacceptable.

7.   Describe an experience when you felt it necessary to limit annoying or un-acceptable behavior on the part of your client. State your reasons for thinking the intervention was necessary and evaluate your intervention. Include the client's reaction to your intervention. Relate your intervention to the client's ability to accept himself and to accept you. How did the experience you describe affect your opinions and feelings about the client?

8.   Describe an experience when you felt it unnecessary or unwise to limit annoying or unacceptable behavior on the part of your client. State your reasons for feeling that intervention was not necessary. Evaluate the apparent results of your nonintervention. How did the experience you describe affect your opinions and feelings about the client?

9.   Describe any of your characteristics that your client has described as being undesirable and give his reasons for his opinion. Include the client's ability to communicate his opinion clearly and tactfully.

Have you limited your behavior in view of the client's expressed opinion? State your reasons for complying or not complying with his opinion.

How did you help the client use the expression of his opinion so that in a similar situation with other people his behavior and expressions might be accepted?

10. How have you protected your client's individuality while helping him to accept common social norms?

11. Describe any differences between the social and cultural values you hold and those of your client.

12. Describe an experience when your client seemed to be testing your determination to maintain the contract between you. Include your response to the testing situation and the results of your response.

13.   Describe an incident when you offered advice to your client. Include the client's reaction to your advice.

Evaluate the results of your giving advice. Include suggestions for change.

14.   When is advice preferable to the use of problem-solving skills?

15.   Why do you continue to maintain the contract if your client appears to wish it broken?

16.   Why do you think the client may wish to break the contract?

INSTRUCTOR'S COMMENTS

CHAPTER 8

Self-Image

During the long process of growth and development, the individual acquires an assessment of himself, derived from the expressions and behavior of people in his environment and from his own experiences with his body and with his activities. When the expressed opinions of others are unanimous, he is likely, at least in his early years, to accept them without question. These opinions, then, become his own assessment of who he is, what he is, what he is worth, what he can and may accomplish, and what he is unable to accomplish. He derives a concept of what he looks like, what his body parts are, where they are, and how he may use them partly through his own observation and experimentation and partly from the expressions of those around him. In this manner he may acquire either a realistic view or a grossly distorted image, both of himself as a person and of his body as it appears to others. The cold, wet, hungry baby whose cry for relief from discomfort is frequently unanswered may acquire a feeling that he is not worth much because, if he were, someone would minister to his needs. Similarly, the adult who, in time of need, asks for help and is ignored may feel that he is of little value. The baby who is neglected in infancy may continue to experience similar reactions throughout childhood so that his feelings of being "nobody," or worse, "nothing," are reinforced.

Many other characteristics are similarly acquired. He may learn that he is "bad" if he becomes dirty, or if he is noisy, or if he runs away. He may also learn that he is fat, or skinny, or ugly, or awkward. Sometimes a statement that is meant in a positive way may have a negative impact. For example, a child is told that he is "just like his father. He is very intelligent, but clumsy with tools." The superficial intent may be to praise the child's intellectual capacity but he may acquire an image of himself as lacking in manual dexterity. Unable to make his own appraisal of himself, he may be forced to accept the impressions of others.

When the child leaves the family group, he is likely to be presented with a conflicting version of his body or self-image. The task of reconciling one view with another may cause difficulty in maintaining an integrated image of himself.

Correcting the distortions may be done from consensual validation and from re-peated experiences that deny the distortion, particularly in respect to ability to function.

The child who has learned from adoring parents that he is superior to others faces a serious problem when he interacts with his peers who may be intolerant of such an attitude.

Many individuals express ideas about themselves that are obvious distortions. A client may say that he is stupid or that he is a genius. He may say that he has no ability to do anything and that he is worthless. All such statements reflect his image of himself as he has learned it from others.

The nurse must attempt to determine how the client views himself so that she may help him use his capabilities realistically, correct a faulty self-image, and be assured of his intrinsic worth.

GUIDE TO ASSESSING THE CLIENT'S SELF-IMAGE

Body Image

1. How does the client describe his appearance?

2. Compare the client's description of himself with your description of him.

3. Describe any gross distortions present in the client's description. Does the client use his body parts in such a way to indicate that he has a distorted body image? If so, describe the behavior and evaluate the meaning of the behavior in relation to the body image.

4. How does the client describe your appearance?

5. Compare the client's description of you with your own image of yourself.

6. Ask a friend to describe your appearance. Compare the three descriptions, yours, your client's, and your friend's, for similarities and dissimilarities. Which description is correct?

7. If the client has a distorted image of his body, can you account for his acquiring such a view?

8. How does the client attempt to validate his body image? Does his attempt at validation result in his changing or maintaining his body image?

9. When your client has a distorted body image which he attempts to prove, will he accept a difference in view? Suggest means of helping the client acquire a realistic body image.

Self-Image

1. List statements made by the client that indicate his opinion of his worth or worthlessness.

2. Compare the client's statement of worth with your assessment of him.

3. Compare the client's statement of worth with those of his relatives.

4. Compare the client's statement of worth with those of professional personnel with whom he has contact.

5. Describe the means the client uses to validate his opinion of his worth or worthlessness.

6. If your assessment of the client's worth is different from that of other people in his environment, validate your assessment by describing experiences that helped form your opinion.

7. Compare your experiences with those of the people in your client's environment who disagree with you. How do you explain the differences?

8. Suggest plans to correct the faulty self-image. Include your reasons for desiring the correction, how you will intervene, and when you will intervene.

9. List statements by the client that indicate his opinion of your worth.

10. Compare the client's opinion of your worth with your own opinion.

11. Suggest reasons why the client's opinion of your worth may be different than your assessment. If you plan to intervene in his opinion of you, state your reasons for so doing and describe the means you intend to use to bring about a change in his opinion.

12. List statements made by your client describing himself in the following roles:

    a. As a child with his parents

    b. As a school child

    c. As a spouse

    d. As a parent himself

    e. As a member of the community

    f. As a church or nonchurch member

g.   As a workman

h.   As a client with a stress problem

12.   Describe any discrepancies, of which you are aware, in the client's self-image in the preceding roles. How do you know the discrepancies are real? Describe your source of information.

13.   Describe any reasons for these discrepancies. Explain your source of information concerning the reasons for the discrepancies.

14.   Summarize briefly the major distortions of body and self-image that your client has expressed.

INSTRUCTOR'S COMMENTS

CHAPTER 9

Perception of Reality

The decisions which the individual makes to produce his behavior are based on his perception of reality. No two people ever perceive any situation in exactly the same manner. Therefore, the perception of reality, like mental health and mental illness, varies on a continuum from a recognizably highly distorted perception as seen in the psychotic to the reasonably accurate (though subject to variation) perception of the "well-adjusted" individual. The perception of reality of the mentally healthy client who may be in a transient stress, or even the mentally healthy individual who is not under stress, must be assessed as carefully as that of the mentally ill client, since it is from this perception that he will decide his course of action. The nurse, therefore, must consider her own perception of reality realizing that, though it may differ from her client's, neither of them is either right or wrong. In fact, the individual experiencing stress, or even the psychotic, may perceive accurately events that are hidden from the nurse or of which, because of her low level of anxiety, she is simply unaware.

The mentally ill have varying degrees of difficulty, as do the mentally healthy, in determining that which is real and that which is unreal. But in the case of the mentally ill person, the ability to maintain the boundary between the unconscious and the conscious mind has become so weakened that much dissociated material becomes mixed with observed reality, and he is unable to differentiate that which is commonly considered real and that which is dissociated and distorted. He responds to voices that are the creation of his own unconscious. His interpretation of and response to the behavior of others and to objects in his environment may depend on reasoning based on faulty perception. His ability to use consensual validation is thus limited not only by his estrangement from other people but also by his distortion of what he does perceive.

Much behavior that the nurse observes and finds unaccountable can be explained, at least in part, when she is able to understand how the client views himself, his environment, and his place in that environment. The nurse who has gained the trust and acceptance of a mentally ill client may be one of the few links between the world of reality and the world of unreality in which the client exists. It is her task to attempt to lead the client gently and slowly toward reality, realizing that the pain and suffering of the client may be so severe that he will not make the journey.

The client who is in a transient state of stress or who, while not psychotic, is experiencing an emotional difficulty, is likely to present a perception of reality that is quite varied. In areas unrelated to his major difficulty, his perception may be reasonable accurate. In those instances in which he experiences such severe stress that his anxiety level causes him to selectively inattend, his perception will be distorted.

In whatever situation the nurse finds herself, whether it be with the emotionally untroubled, with the client who is under stress, or with the severely psychotic, an understanding of his perception of reality will be necessary to an understanding of his behavior.

GUIDE FOR PERCEPTION OF REALITY

Perception of Self

1. From the data used to describe the client's self-image, briefly restate the client's perception of reality concerning himself. Indicate with an asterisk areas which you consider distorted.

    a. Body image

    b. Self-image

2.   If your client is psychotic, describe any indications that his perception of himself is unreal, such as: "I am a ghost." "I am not alive."

3.   Indicate your response to the client's statement of unreality, your reasons for your response, and the client's reaction.

4.   Evaluate your intervention and suggest an alternate means of intervention.

5.   Describe any apparent reason or cause for the presence of the feeling of unreality. Include your source of information concerning the possible cause and theoretical knowledge that supports your opinion.

6. Describe your plan of intervention to encourage the client to adopt a more realistic self-image if you think it is desirable to do so. Include your reasons for thinking intervention is desirable. If you think intervention is not desirable, state your reasons for your conclusion.

Perception of Other People

1. Describe the client's usual response to most people whom he meets on a casual basis, e.g., friendly, hostile, warm, cold. Indicate any reasons he has stated for his responses.

2. Compare the client's usual approach to others to his first approach to you. If there is a difference, explain what the difference is and why it occurred.

3. Describe the client's perception of significant people in his most comfortable milieu. Compare it to your perception of these people and indicate any apparent reasons for any discrepancies between your perceptions.

4. Describe the client's perception of significant people in his most uncomfortable milieu. Compare it to your perception of these people and indicate any apparent reasons for discrepancies between your perceptions.

5. If your client appears to be hallucinating, describe the hallucination as the client relates it. Include your understanding of the basic meaning of the hallucination.

6. If the client recognizes that he hallucinates, describe his understanding of what an hallucination is and how he acquired this knowledge. How and when does he recognize that he is hallucinating?

7. Identify conditions which you have observed cause your client to hallucinate.

8. Identify any means being used to alleviate the hallucinatory state. If no attempt at active intervention is being made, explain.

9. Identify any means that you have used to intervene in the hallucinatory state. Include your reasons for intervening and the results. If you were not successful, suggest an alternate means.

10. Describe an experience in which your client misinterpreted the behavior of others. Include your own interpretation of the behavior in question.

11.   What was your response to the client's misinterpretation? State your reasons for your response and the client's reaction to the response.

12.   Evaluate your intervention and suggest an alternate means of intervention.

13.   Describe your means of gaining understanding of the behavior that your client misinterpreted. How did you validate your own interpretation of the behavior which was observed by you and your client?

14.   What do you think was the probable cause of the misinterpretations by your client? State what evidence you have of the probable cause. Include theoretical knowledge to support your opinion.

Perception of the Environment

1. Describe the client's perception of the world in general, i.e., "O.K.," "not too bad," "a troubled mess," "in danger of holocaust." Include the means he used to make his perceptions and his responses to what he perceives.

2. Describe your client's perception of his immediate neighborhood and compare it to your own perception.

CLIENT	NURSE
a. Socio-economic level	a.
b. Safety	b.
c. Comfort, convenience	c.
d. Racial, ethnic, cultural factors	d.

3. Indicate the means your client uses to make his perceptions and his response to his perceptions.

4. Indicate the means you used to make your perceptions. Explain any discrepancies between your perceptions and the client's.

5. Assess the validity to himself of the client's perceptions by observing his responses to his environment. For example, if the client states his neighborhood is a safe one, yet will not go out alone because he is afraid, his perception is not valid. He may believe what he states as perceiving but his nonverbal behavior contradicts, or makes invalid, his statement.

6. List any statements made by the client that indicate he perceives himself as a part of his neighborhood or as alienated from it.

7. Describe your client's perception of his family in general, e.g., "typical," "different," "better than most," "horrible." Compare it to your own perception and explain any discrepancies between your perception and the client's.

8. Describe your client's perception of his family's role and status in the immediate neighborhood. Compare his assessment with yours and indicate the means each of you has used to·make the perceptions. Indicate and explain discrepancies in the two assessments.

9. Describe your client's perception of his family in particular, such as cold, chaotic, safe, protective. Indicate the basis of his perceptions. Compare his perceptions and yours, indicate and explain any discrepancies.

10. List any statements made by the client that indicate he perceives himself as a part of the family or as alienated from it.

11. Describe the client's perception of his status and role in the family. Compare his assessment with yours and indicate the basis of your perceptions. Indicate and explain any discrepancies in the two assessments.

Result of Defective Perception of Reality

1. Describe behavior you have observed that resulted from the client's failure to perceive or interpret reality adequately or accurately.

2. What does the client gain from misinterpreting or failing to perceive reality?

3. What does he lose by his failure?

4. What purpose does the unreality serve?

Summary

1. Summarize briefly the client's difficulties in perceiving or interpreting reality.

INSTRUCTOR'S COMMENTS

CHAPTER 10

Levels of Functioning

Erik Erikson describes eight stages of development through which man passes from birth to death.[1] Each stage must be partially completed before the next is attempted, and if the individual is to function eventually as a mature, mentally healthy adult, he must complete each level to a measurable extent. When these states are not successfully completed, the individual is handicapped in establishing an adequate relationship with himself and others. His ability to adjust to his environment is thereby limited. The person who is mentally ill may be handicapped in all of the stages of development or only in some of them. In order to help the client to learn healthy ways of relating to himself, to others, and to his environment, it is necessary to assess his level of functioning.

Assessment of a client's level of functioning is a complex task that involves observing and then interpreting verbal and nonverbal behavior. No assessment should be made without sufficient data. The most mature well adjusted adult may occasionally regress under stress to a very early level of development, yet such regression is hardly indicative of his usual functioning. The nurse is concerned in making her assessment with the level on which the client customarily functions or with a particular phase of development which may be incomplete.

Some verbal responses and certain nonverbal behavior are characteristic of the various levels. The following chart indicates a few of the customary responses.

---

[1] Erikson, Erik H.; *Childhood and Society*. New York: W. W. Norton Co., 1964.

Level	Verbal Expressions	Nonverbal Behavior
Trust vs.	"I believe you" "I can tell you about . . ." "You will help me I know." "You are my friend."	Sharing time, opinions, emotions, experiences. Asking for help with the expectation of receiving it. Accepting help from others comfortably.
Mistrust	"I am afraid of you." "I can't tell you about anything." "You cheat." "Stool pigeon."	Refusing to share time, opinions, emotions, experiences. Unable to accept help. Confining conversation to superficialities. Controlling behavior so that only that which is usually socially approved is exhibited.
Autonomy vs.	"I will." "I won't." "If you want me to, I will this time. Next time, maybe not." "This is my opinion. What is yours?" "I can wait."	Accepting group rules but expressing dissent when it is felt. Accepting leadership role when appropriate. Expressing own opinion. Accepting postponement of wish gratification easily.
Shame and Doubt	"My opinion doesn't count." "I never know the answers." "Whatever you say . . ." "I don't want to hear what you say. I must be right." "I should do that."	Overly concerned with being clean. Not maintaining own opinion when opposed. Failing to express needs. Maintaining own opinion despite adequate proof to the contrary. Unable to wait. Hoarding. Soiling. Being vindictive.
Initiative vs.	"Let me try!" "What is this? How does it work?" "Where does that road go?"	Exploring. Starting new projects with eagerness. Expressing curiosity. Being original.
Guilt	"I am afraid to start." "You go first and I will follow." "I am ashamed to make a mistake."	Imitating others rather than developing ideas independently. Expressing a great deal of embarrassment over a small mistake.

Level	Verbal Expressions	Nonverbal Behavior
Industry vs. *Inferiority*	"I am working on this. When it is done, I will start that." "I like to be busy." "Group projects are fun." "I can't work with other people." "I have a lot of things going but nothing finished."	Completing a task once it has been started. Working well with others. Using time effectively. Not completing any set tasks. Not contributing to the work of others. Not organizing work.
Identity vs. *Identity diffusion*	"I am going to be a nurse." "I believe in these principles." "I think that mothers should do this and fathers do that." "I am on my own." "What do these things mean to me?" "I don't know who I am." "Where am I going?" "Is it better to be male or female?" "I don't know what I mean."	Establishing relationships with same sex and then with opposite sex. Planning realistically for future roles. Re-examining values. Asserting independence. Trying various roles. Failing to differentiate roles or goals in life. Failing to assume responsibility for directing own behavior. Imitating others indiscriminately. Accepting values of others without question.
Intimacy vs. *Isolation*	"We are very close friends." "I love John." "He chased me until I caught him." "I am a loner." "I don't need anyone." "I don't care about anyone."	Establishing a close and intense relationship with another person. Acting out and accepting sexual behavior as desirable. Remaining alone. Not seeking out others for companionship or help. Avoiding establishing contacts with members of opposite sex. Avoiding sex role by attempting to remain nondescript in mannerisms and clothing.

Level	Verbal Expressions	Nonverbal Behavior
Generativity vs.	"John and I agreed to have two children." "He has his work and I have mine. Together we make a team." "I enjoy teaching kindergarten. The children are so happy to learn."	Willingness to share work with another. Accepting interdependence. Guiding others. Establishing a priority of needs to recognize both self and others.
Self-absorption	"You worked all night? Well, it's your turn to care for the baby. I'm going out."	Not listening to others because of need to talk about oneself. Showing concern only for oneself despite needs of others.
Integrity vs.	"Life has been good to me." "My son will carry on my name when I am gone." "I can't do what I used to, but I do enjoy other things." "I have left my mark in the world." "I enjoy talking about current events." "What is death?"	Using past experience to guide others. Accepting new ideas. Maintaining skill suitable to physical condition. Maintaining productivity in some area. Accepting limitations. Exploring a philosophy of living and dying.
Despair	"I am no use to anyone." "Every one is gone—my family, my friends. What is the sense of living?" "I can't do anything." "Everything I did is gone now. Why did I bother and work?" "These new ways are no good."	Crying. Being apathetic and listless. Not developing any interests beyond a few routine activities. Not accepting changes. Limiting interpersonal contacts. Denying the inevitable nonexistence. Demanding unnecessary help and attention.

In the following check list, the eight stages of development described by Erikson are listed. Select data from five of your recordings to complete the check list. Count the number of expressions by your client that are indicative of the various levels of development. Total the numbers. From the totals, make an assessment of the areas in which your client has difficulty functioning and the levels in which he apparently does not function at all. See the following example.

Level of Functioning	Recordings					Total
	1	2	3	4	5	
Trust vs.	0	1	0	0	1	2
Mistrust	3	4	3	1	4	15

Assessment:

The client has difficulty in the first stage of development. He expressed trust twice and mistrust 15 times in the period of the five selected interviews.

CHECK LIST FOR LEVELS OF FUNCTIONING

Level of Functioning	Recordings					Total
	1	2	3	4	5	
Trust vs. Mistrust						
Autonomy vs. Shame and Doubt						
Initiative vs. Guilt						
Industry vs. Inferiority						
Identity vs. Identity Diffusion						
Intimacy vs. Isolation						
Generativity vs. Self-Absorption						
Integrity vs. Despair						

GUIDE FOR ASSESSMENT

1. From your recordings and completed check list of the levels of functioning, list the stages of development which your client seems to have completed successfully. Describe three experiences or verbal comments to validate your conclusion.

2. List levels of development in which the client is having difficulty, and describe three experiences or verbal comments indicative of the problem areas.

3. List stages of development which your client does not give any indication of having reached.

INSTRUCTOR'S COMMENTS

PART II

THEORETICAL BACKGROUND

CHAPTER 11

Assessment and Statement of the Problem

The orientation or beginning phase of the nurse-client relationship will vary in length. It consists primarily of a period during which the nurse collects the data she needs while simultaneously establishing a relationship of trust and acceptance between herself and the client. When this phase is completed, the nurse may find herself with a plethora of data and problems which combine to make her feel confused and not sure of what she is doing or what she should do next.

The purpose of this section of the workbook is to arrange data in a coherent fashion to help the nurse set some priorities. The student will find that in completing the guides, she will necessarily be repeating much information that she has already provided. However, the repetitiveness of the procedure serves to provide a different focus in many instances, as well as preparing the nurse to use all of the data she has in an orderly manner. For example, early in the workbook the nurse was observing communication skills. At this time, she might well have thought that the basis of the client's problems lay in his inability to communicate. Had she developed a plan of care at this point, her focus would have been on improving communication. At a later period, she was assessing the client's self-image. Then she thought that the poor self-image was the major problem and this would be the focus of a care plan. By assembling in one area all the available data, the nurse will gain an overall picture of her client which should provide the information she needs to develop a workable plan with some measure of success.

Having collected and analyzed sufficient data, the nurse will identify a specific problem. Once the problem is identified, she will need to acquire specific theoretical material to give her an understanding of the dynamics involved. She can then proceed, in conjunction with the client, to explore the basic problem fully, and to devise some means by which the client can remove, alleviate, or live with the problem in some degree of comfort.

It is not the purpose of this workbook to discuss a specific theoretical approach to the maintenance of mental health, prevention of mental illness, or treatment and rehabilitation of the mentally ill. It is obvious, however, that to work consistently in a goal-directed manner, rather than to be subject to the whim of the moment, the student will need to have basic theories related to personality development and psychopathology well in mind. The student will need to organize theoretical material she may have gained from several sources to form an integrated background which will clarify the observations she has been making, and assist her to develop a nursing care plan consistent with her theoretical beliefs and the observations of her client and his milieus.

The first decision the nurse will have to make is to determine what is mental health. Students eventually become bored with attempting to make what is actually a nearly impossible determination. However, the student needs some standards by which to make judgments concerning adaptive and maladaptive behavior.

It is suggested that the student develop a very general list of what are ordinarily considered attributes of mental health. She can then develop a second list of what she considers to be the attributes of mental health which would be appropriate to her specific client within his unique life situation. The purpose of the two lists is to help the student bridge some of the cultural and socio-economic differences that make the definition of mental health so vague. The first list is a very general one and helps provide a base. The second one usually prevents the nurse from assessing behavior as maladaptive when in actual fact, given the client's unique milieus, his behavior is adaptive. It also prevents her from trying to encourage the formation of behavior which in some circumstances is adaptive but which would actually be maladaptive for the client. An example of such a situation is described by a student who initially made a home visit as a follow-up to a medical emergency. She gave the following report:

> The family consists of three adults, two of whom work in nearby factories, and the third, the medical patient who maintains the household. The client described her pleasure in cooking and cleaning and keeping "things just so" for her working brother and sister. Further conversation indicated that she never left the home, not even to grocery shop. The other sister and brother left the home only to work. Other behavior indicated that the working brother and sister depended on the client as though she were a mother. There were also other indications of eccentric behavior. The nurse described the milieu as being pleasant, warm, and relaxed, apparently as a result of the efforts of the client. However, stability was being maintained at a heavy price. To all appearances, the client was suppressing desires for greater contact with the outside world in order to keep peace within the family.

In assessing this situation, the nurse decided that greater independence should gradually be encouraged so that the client would have greater contact away from home and the other sister and brother could become less dependent. The nurse made several attempts to put her plan into practice and, with increasing familiarity with the family, eventually discovered that, had her plan been implemented, she probably would have had three psychotic individuals with whom to work. The relationship between the three family members was one of nearly forty years' duration and, therefore, firmly established. The stress of the medical emergency had pointed out the depths of the needs of all three members.

Further visits eventually brought to light that the client had developed various ways of reducing her isolation and gaining some personal time even over some rather mild objections by the other two. She had several hobbies which she followed in the home setting and she also managed to maintain a small circle of friends who visited her despite the fact that she could not visit them. Any activity being carried out on the street outside she watched with avid interest, even while the nurse was visiting. Her comment was, "You have to make your own fun in life. If I didn't work around my problems and fit things in somehow I guess I'd go crazy, although every time I sit down to go crazy, someone wants a cup of tea and I don't have time." This rather astute lady had come to terms with her milieu and, although it is maladaptive from some viewpoints, given the unique family circumstances which could probably not have been changed, her behavior was actually adaptive. One does not expect a cardiac patient compensated by medication to climb Mt. Everest. Neither should one expect a similar miracle from the individual who has an emotional problem. Complete active involvement in the community and dealing with great stress may be as impossible goals for some as climbing the mountain is for others.

Statement of the problem which has caused the client to need help may or may not be in terms of a psychiatric diagnosis. In any event, the nurse needs to have a clear definition of a problem. Once the problem has been stated, the usual causative factors identified within the theoretical framework which the nurse is using must be elaborated. It is usually of value to explore many theoretical bases rather than cling to one area. Many times, ideas from one theory can be incorporated within another to increase the nurse's understanding of possible causes of the client's difficulties.

The cause of events likely to accompany problems such as the client's, and the usual means of remediation required to alleviate or reduce the problem, are next considered. Here again the nurse is wise to consult different theorists to give her a complete picture of present day thinking. It is necessary to identify both psychiatric and nursing practices used in treatment so that her particular care plan will be consistent with whatever psychiatric regime has been augmented, and so that she herself may make valuable contributions in terms of her observations and her care.

ASSESSMENT OF THE STRENGTHS AND WEAKNESSES OF THE CLIENT

Directions: Using the data assembled in Part I and your interaction notes, complete the following guide to help you assess your client's areas of strengths and weaknesses. Include verbatim data and actual experiences to validate your observations.

Area	Strengths	Weaknesses
A. Communication		
1. Clarity		
2. Accuracy		
3. Preciseness		
4. Descriptive ability		
5. Use of concrete terms		
6. Use of abstract terms		
7. Use of logical associations		
B. Perception of Reality		
1. Self-image		

Area	Strengths	Weaknesses
2. Body image		
3. Interpretation of environment		
4. Interpretation of others in environment		
C. *Ability to Function* 1. Body care a. Personal hygiene b. Maintenance of body functions		
2. Observance of common safety needs		
3. Use of manual skill		

Area	Strengths	Weaknesses
4. Use of intellectual skills		
5. Use of skill in interpersonal relations a. with relatives		
b. with peers		
c. with authority figures		
d. with you		
D. *Levels of development* 1. Trust		
2. Autonomy		
3. Initiative		

Area	Strengths	Weaknesses
4. Industry		
5. Identity		
6. Intimacy		
7. Generativity		
8. Integrity		

ASSESSMENT OF STRENGTHS AND WEAKNESSES OF NURSE

Directions: Use of data from Part I and your interaction notes to complete the following items.

Area	Strengths	Weaknesses
A. *Communications* 1. Clarity		
2. Accuracy		
3. Conciseness		
4. Encouragement of client's verbalization		
5. Recognition of client's difficulties in communication		
6. Recognition of own difficulties in communication		

Area	Strengths	Weaknesses
7. Recognition of recurrent themes		
8. Ability to pursue area of concern		
B. *Nonverbal Behavior* 1. Ability to listen with attention		
2. Ability to control nonverbal expressions of emotions		
3. Ability to maintain or use silence		
4. Ability to control undesirable gestures or mannerisms		

Area	Strengths	Weaknesses
C. *Establishment of Nurse-Client Relationship*		
1. Approach		
2. Observation of client problems		
3. Understanding of client problems		
4. Observation of own problems		
5. Understanding of own problems		
6. Establishment of trust		
7. Evaluation of nurse-client interaction		

Area	Strengths	Weaknesses
D. *Specific Characteristics and Their Effect on Interactions* 1. Age		
2. Past experience		
3. Unique assets or handicaps		

ASSESSMENT OF THE MILIEUS

Directions: Using data assembled in Part I and your interaction notes, complete the following guide to assess strengths and weaknesses of the client's milieus.

The Comfortable Milieu

Area	Strengths	Weaknesses
1. Physical needs	1.	1.
2. Physical comfort	2.	2.
3. Psychological comfort	3.	3.
4. Personal space	4.	4.
5. Personal time	5.	5.
6. Possibility of change	6.	6.
7. Greatest asset	7.	7.
8. Greatest weakness	8.	8.

The Uncomfortable Milieu

Area	Strengths	Weaknesses
1. Physical needs	1.	1.
2. Physical comfort	2.	2.
3. Psychological comfort	3.	3.
4. Personal space	4.	4.
5. Personal time	5.	5.
6. Possibility of change	6.	6.
7. Greatest asset	7.	7.
8. Greatest weakness	8.	8.

STATEMENT OF THE PROBLEM

Directions: From the data organized so far in Part II, complete the following questions:

1. State what you observe as the client's major problem and include the reasons for your decision.

2. State what you observe as minor problems which contribute to the major problem. Indicate the manner in which they affect the major problem.

3. State what the client considers to be his major problem and include his reasons for his selection.

4. State what the client considers to be minor problems and include his reasons for so thinking.

5. If there is a discrepancy between your selection of a major problems and the client's, indicate what you consider to be the cause of the discrepancy.

INSTRUCTOR'S COMMENTS

CHAPTER 12

Theoretical Approach

1. State the particular theoretical approach you intend to use, e.g., psycho-analytical, behavioristic, eclectic.

Answer the following questions in accordance with your choice of theory.

2. List attributes indicative of mental health.

3. List attributes indicative of your client's mental health considering his unique life and life experiences.

4. Describe in detail the theoretical considerations of your client's stated problem in relation to etiology, symptomatology, usual progression of problem, prognosis, and treatment.

5.   Describe professional treatment and nonprofessional help the client has received in the past for his problem.

    a.   Professional treatment

    b.   Nonprofessional help

6.   Describe any nursing care the client has received.

7. Describe the effects of treatment or help received.

    a. Professional treatment

    b. Nonprofessional help

    c. Nursing

Bibliography Used for Your Theoretical Approach:

INSTRUCTOR'S COMMENTS

CHAPTER 13

Plan of
Nursing Care

In developing a plan of care, the nurse must remember that she cannot establish goals for the client. The client establishes his own goals which will be compatible with his life style and situation. The nurse's purpose in developing a care plan is to provide for herself a basis from which she can provide guidance to the client.

The nurse encourages the client to identify certain behaviors as adaptive or maladaptive. She may further encourage him to desire certain behaviors or eliminate others in order to help him adjust more comfortably to his situation. She may then attempt to create a climate, either within the nurse-client relationship or within a specific milieu, where the client may practice changed behavior. It is wise to remember how painfully slow behavioral change may occur. An orderly, step by step plan will help maintain progress.

The nurse must make use of the practical situation or milieu in which her client lives so that she does not doom her plan to failure by developing unrealistic, unattainable goals before she even gets started. As stated earlier, change in the client may be met by resistance from those in the milieu. Some milieus are nearly impossible to change and must be accepted as just that. On the other hand, many times a change in the milieu is what encourages the client to change behavior.

The plan of care must be based on a solid theoretical framework and not on "intuition" or "this worked before". The theoretical framework, as a means to explain and predict behaviors, will assist the nurse in maintaining a reasoned, consistent approach and help her to avoid falling prey to feelings of hopelessness and inadequacy.

The plan of care, like the rest of the nurse-client relationship, is concerned with the nurse and her behavior as factors that will influence desired results.

GUIDE FOR PLAN OF NURSING CARE

1. List behaviors which you have observed in your client which are ordinarily considered maladaptive.

2. Of the above behaviors, which ones are adaptive to his particular milieu?

3. Of the above maladaptive behaviors observed, list those which can realistically be changed.

4. Describe the steps it would be necessary for the client to take in order to change his behavior.

5. Describe changes in the milieu which must be made in order for the client to change his behavior.

6. If change in the milieu is to precede behavioral change in the client, describe the process by which the milieu will be altered.

7. Construct a plan of care, using the model provided on pages 177 and 178.

8. Using the theoretical framework you have selected, describe how you expect your nursing care plan will affect the dynamics of the client's personality structure.

Adaptive Behavior To Be Strengthened	Means To Be Used To Strengthen Behavior		Contributing Elements	
			Strengths	Weaknesses
		Client		
		Nurse		
		Milieu		

Maladaptive Behavior To Be Lessened	Means To Be Used To Decrease Maladaptive Behavior	Contributing Elements		
			Strengths	*Weaknesses*
		Client		
		Nurse		
		Milieu		

INSTRUCTOR'S COMMENTS

PART III

IMPLEMENTATION OF THE PLAN OF CARE

CHAPTER 14

Implementation as a Learning Process

The nursing care plan basically is a unit in a learning program. Problem solving skills have been used to collect data and identify areas of difficulty which prevent the client from living in some degree of comfort. In order for the client to function ideally in maximum comfort he must be able to perform in an interdependent fashion. This means that he needs a realistic knowledge of his strengths and weaknesses and those of others in his milieu. He needs a realistic knowledge of his milieu, how it affects him and how he affects it. He needs to know the effects of change in any of these areas and how to bring about orderly change if necessary, and using this knowledge he must be able to live so that he can function independently, dependently, or interdependently, as the situation requires. These are all factors which are incorporated in the nursing care plan.

However, to implement the care plan, it will be necessary to help the client not only to learn about himself, other people, his milieus, and the process of change but also to learn how he learns and how he can use his learning. Therefore, the nursing care plan is initiated by using the basic steps in a learning process whether that learning be arithmetic, reading, or changing one's behavior. Frank M. Hewett in *Education of Exceptional Learners*[1] states:

> From the broad psycho-social dimensions of flexibility, sociality, intelligence, and individualization, we turn to consideration of dimensions related to learning (in the classroom)—attention, response, exploratory, social, and mastery. These dimensions describe levels of learning competence that are essential for success [in school].

---

[1] Hewett, Frank. *Education of Exceptional Learners.* Boston, Allyn and Bacon, 1974, p. 219.

Attention and Response

The nurse, in adopting this sequence, may think that she has already accomplished at least the first two steps of attention and response. That is, both she and her client have listened (attended) to each other in order to identify necessary data, and both have responded to each other by establishing their relationship so that the working phase, based on trust and acceptance, has begun. While it may be true that the levels of attention and response have been met concerning the relationship in general, the nursing care plan focuses not on a general relationship, but on a specific area of difficulty. Therefore, the nurse begins the implementation of her care plan by starting at the beginning level of attention.

Referring back to Chapter 11, the nurse will observe a question relative to agreement between herself and the client concerning the nature of the basic problem. If disagreement exists, it must be resolved. The client is not likely to be motivated to work on a problem he considers unimportant. The nurse, also, is likely to be frustrated by what she may identify as denial by the client of his actual difficulties. If agreement does exist, the nurse still needs to start her care plan at the attention level. It may only be necessary to recapitulate in a matter of a few moments what both she and the client have agreed on as the major difficulty to be attacked. The mutual discussion will move both nurse and client through the first two levels of attention and response.

However, the attainment of the first level of attention is particularly difficult when the client has a short attention span, as in emotionally disturbed children or adult clients with hypomania. Lack of attention will be identified easily by the nurse as the client constantly jumps from one subject to another, possibly dropping a few cues as to his basic problem but quickly shifting to a safe topic of irrelevant conversation. At this point, in order to begin implementing the care plan, the nurse may need to set firm limits with the client in order first to gain his attention.

Setting limits can be a serious problem for some nurses. They fear that not to allow the client to ramble about whatever he chooses is to breach the contract. After all, the interview time is for the client to talk about, or not talk about, whatever he chooses. To deny him this privilege is to reduce his independence. Granted that the client does have the right to his independence, the contract also states that the relationship is to be a therapeutic one. Therefore, the nurse must decide that in order to meet the major aspect of being therapeutic or helping, she must indeed reduce the client's inattentiveness, which is probably pathological, by setting a limit. This does not mean that she can maintain the client's attention for the entire time of the interview. She may consider herself successful if she can maintain attention for only five minutes during a fifty-minute hour in some instances. The problem of attentiveness may actually be the major difficulty stated in her care plan. Success will be interpreted as gaining and increasing the attentive level with some response on the part of the client.

Attentiveness may be limited if the client is so severely depressed that his thinking is totally self-centered and he is unable to move his thoughts from a repetitive sequence of guilt, remorse, and hopelessness. The same may be true of the autistic child or the hallucinating schizophrenic. However, the possibility exists that the client does indeed attend but is unable to attain the second level of response. This is particularly true of the client who is in a catatonic stupor, apparently totally unaware of anything outside himself, yet who, as he becomes well, recounts in detail many events to which he did attend but was unable to make a response.

Another common factor that seems to prevent some nurses from setting limits is the fear of alienating the client or destroying his sense of trust and acceptance. In actual fact, the firm setting of a reasonable limit appears to tell the client that he can indeed trust the nurse, that she is willing to help even at the price of discomfort to both of them, and that she accepts him in spite of what she indicates by the limit setting as unacceptable behavior.

The level of attention is best described as a period when the client and the nurse are listening to each other, observing, and cataloguing events as they have occurred in the past or during the relationship. The level of response usually accompanies the level of attention closely. The nurse and the client react or respond to what they are observing. It is necessary in a therapeutic nurse-client relationship to attend to the response level as well as to other events occurring at the attention level. In other words, the nurse must assess not only to what the client attends, what he observes, of what he is aware (the attention level), but also how he responds to these observations (the response level). Much of the nurse's work to this point has been concerned with these two levels.

Exploratory Level

In implementing the nursing care plan the nurse, after establishing agreement or stating a mutual identification of a problem area, moves into the exploratory level. This is an exciting time for both nurse and client. Usually the identification of a problem gives a feeling of success to both, a sense of direction and purpose. During the exploratory period, the nurse and client together examine themselves and the milieu, searching for means of removing the difficulty. The nurse, from her care plan, has already reached some conclusions, but exploring various avenues of approach with the client not only is likely to result in modifying her plan, but also provides her with a golden opportunity to teach problem-solving skills that will insure future success in similar ventures by her client. To teach problem-solving skills is to maintain the nurse-client relationship in perpetuity. It is perhaps the greatest benefit of the relationship. While the exploratory period may be exciting for some clients, many clients will be limited by the anxiety provoked by moving from an accustomed rut. Other clients will be even more seriously limited by a lack of knowledge of what help is available simply because they may have spent years in an impoverished environment. The exploratory period is chiefly a looking around, an identification of physical objects, identifying means to an end.

Social Level

The next level, that of a social dimension, is probably the most anxiety-provoking for the emotionally disturbed, and possibly the area in which they have the least understanding. The social level focuses on personal and interpersonal relations, societal factors, and ordinarily acceptable social behavior, all of which may be a complete enigma to many people. The nurse may have little difficulty until her client reaches this level. For example, a nurse working with a client who had an exceptionally high intellectual and educational background discovered he had great difficulty in acquiring work other than that of an unskilled laborer. After a thorough completion of the exploratory level, the client discovered a job opening suitable for his requirements and proceeded to apply for the job with his usual lack of success. In discouragement he returned to the nurse and together they recapped his job interview. He had introduced himself, stated his educational background, and then informed his prospective employer that he would report for work the next day, that he would receive a specific salary and vacation time and be promoted within a year. The nurse had failed to assess his social level, unaware that he had difficulties in understanding that everyone did not realize his tremendous potential, and that he lacked basic social knowledge of how to apply for a job.

Many times social competence can best be viewed in a group situation. Obviously, the nurse can assist the client in developing successful interactions with herself, but social relations with a group can be very different. Direct observations by the nurse or observations by other professionals of competence at the social level are necessary. The report by the client is, of course, vital, but it is also biased. A comparison of how he sees his interactions with the nurse's observations may serve to move the client through the social level by helping him "see himself as others see him," by understanding his effect on others, and by understanding their responses.

Many clients from impoverished backgrounds need basic knowledge of simple social skills such as table manners, thank you notes, or what to wear. Role playing or guided experience in controlled situations can provide convenient tools to help acquire these skills. For example, some nurses working with adolescent girls in a slum area guided the girls in providing a "social evening" for the elderly in a community housing project. The purpose of the "social evening" was explained to the elderly who gladly assisted the adolescents as they were guided by the nurses through the social amenities that were completely foreign to them. It was a successful evening for all three groups, the elderly, the adolescents, and the nurses.

Mastery

The final level, mastery, is acquired usually only after much practice. Mastery in learning to walk is acquired only after so many painful falls. The persistence of the year old baby in learning this skill is precisely what the client is likely to need to practice his new behavior. The nurse functions chiefly as an observer, encourager, and listener at this point. As mastery is gradually achieved, the nurse begins to move toward termination by encouraging greater independence by the client. It is always difficult to act as a bystander, particularly if the nurse thinks the client is going to "fall." However, he must fall and learn to pick himself up if mastery is to be achieved. The client who is never allowed to make his mistakes, never learns to deal with failure.

In considering means of implementing the nursing care plan, the nurse's theoretical framework will help determine her guidance. The resulting consistent approach will help keep the client's objective in focus, both for himself and the nurse, as he meets the difficulties inevitable as change approaches. Regression and vacillation are expected accompaniments of the attainment of mastery.

Having made steady progress for a time, the client may enter a period in which he appears neither to progress nor regress. He merely stands still. Many times this represents a solidifying and stabilizing period where newly acquired skills are being integrated permanently into the client's behavioral pattern.

Following the period of rest and consolidation, the client may take the final steps that indicate mastery. Again the nurse will need to remember that there are negative aspects in attaining even a positive goal. These negative aspects may, for a time, intensify, until the goal is finally within reach and the client at long last reaches his objective. One is reminded of the hesitant bridegroom who, two months before his proposed marriage, was most enthusiastic concerning the state of wedded bliss, yet the night before the actual ceremony thought longingly of the carefree days of bachelorhood which he was about to surrender to years of suffering and bondage.

Sometimes the learning which occurs in one area of living will spread and affect another area. For example, the method learned to solve a problem in one milieu can be transferred to another. Another example can be found in the improvement of communication skills which help the client interact more successfully with other people. Improved interactions may in turn lead to an improved work or social situation.

As the client achieves mastery in his own area of difficulty, the nurse is also achieving mastery of nursing skills. Constant evaluation, or attention, responding to her own evaluations, exploring ways of guiding her client, and identifying the social and practical aspects of her functioning should lead her to some degree of mastery of the very complex skills required in therapeutic nursing.

It may be helpful at this point for the student to read the guide to crisis intervention in the following chapter, as much of the material therein is related to implementing the plan of care.

GUIDE FOR IMPLEMENTATION OF CARE PLAN

Directions: Using your recordings, complete the following items.

1. Describe steps of learning that have been used prior to the implementation of your care plan. In response to what situations and with what results were these steps used? Indicate your client's knowledge of these behaviors as steps in the learning process and his ability to use these steps in other learning situations.

2. Describe steps in problem-solving techniques you have used prior to the implementation of your care plan. In response to what situations and with what results were these steps used? Indicate your client's knowledge of problem-solving techniques and his ability to use them.

3. State the major difficulties you have had to date in the attending-responding levels as you attempted to establish a therapeutic relationship. Include your attempts at intervention and the results.

4. Identify difficulties between yourself and your client in reaching agreement as to the area of difficulty in which you will work.

5. State any modifications in the nursing care plan as a result of the above difficulty. Include any changes in the approach to be used by you and your client.

6. Describe the ability of the client to meet the attention level. As you begin to work on the problem about which you and your client agreed include your attempts at inaugurating and maintaining this level and the client's ability to attend.

7. List specific areas in which the client has no difficulty attending.

8. Describe specific areas in which the client does not attend. Indicate any apparent reasons for the inattention, your attempts to gain attention, and the result of your attempts.

9. Describe adaptive responses made by the client to the details of the care plan to which he has been attending.

10. Describe maladaptive responses made by the client to the details of the care plan to which he has been attending. Include your intervention into the maladaptive responses and the results of your intervention.

11. Describe attempts by the client to explore means of attacking his problem. Include any guidance you have provided either in encouraging exploration or as a response to independent exploration by the client.

12.   List all the means the client has explored and found useful to him. Rank them in the client's order of priority, that is, what does he see as most efficacious, what next, and so on to the least useful.

13.   Describe the means by which the client arrived at the decision as to which action to take. Include your response both to the action and to the manner in which he made his decision.

14.   Describe other means available to the client which he did not consider. Why did he not consider the other means? If you intend to bring the means to your client's attention, how will you do so? If you do not, include your reasons for not making the data available.

15.   Describe your client's expectations of the responses of others to his attempts to change his behavior or the milieu.

16. Describe your assessment of the responses likely to occur as a result of changes.

17. Describe any behavior by your client that indicates either a lack of knowledge of customary social behavior or a lack of understanding of the impact his behavior is likely to have on others.

18. Describe intervention on your part to improve the client's level of social knowledge and responsiveness.

19. Describe attempts by the client to prepare others for a change in his behavior or in the milieu so that change can take place in an orderly fashion.

20. Describe attempts on your part to prepare the client for the effects of change. Include his response.

21.   Describe intervention on your part to prepare others for change in the client. Include their responses.

22.   Describe the client's evaluation of his attempts at change.

23.   Describe vacillation or regression by the client as he continues to implement a change in his behavior. Include your response to his behavior.

24.   Describe the client's behavior during a plateau or period when neither progression nor regression appears to be occurring. If the plateau is observed, indicate how long it lasts and what occurred to terminate the plateau.

25.   Describe negative responses by the client or by others that occurred following some behavioral changes that are a result of the implementation of the care plan. Include your response to the negativism.

26.   Describe opportunities available for the client to practice changed behavior. How often can he practice and how effective is his practice?

27.   Describe the client's response to any failures he experienced during his practice toward mastery. Include your feelings about his failures, your response, and why you think he failed.

28.   Describe indications that the client has mastered the changed behavior.

29.   Indicate other potential areas of learning which may occur as a result of his behavioral change.

30.   Describe the client's evaluation of the entire implementation of the care plan.

31.   Describe the evaluation of the client's changed behavior by others in the milieu.

32.   Describe your evaluation of the implementation of the care plan.

33.   If the client's evaluation is unrealistic, state your reasons for thinking so and describe further steps you have taken to verify your own evaluation.

34.   Describe your plans for helping the client develop a realistic self-evaluation.

INSTRUCTOR'S COMMENTS

CHAPTER 15

Crisis Intervention

Crisis intervention is a specialized area in psychiatric–mental health practice. It is included in this workbook, not in the detail required if one were to specialize in this area, but only as it is related to the implementation of the nursing care plan. Implementation of the care plan has been described as a learning process. Learning includes developmental behavioral change. Crisis, as a concomitant part of developmental change, will occur to some degree as the nursing care plan is implemented.

A crisis exists when an individual experiences stress which he is unable to relieve by the use of his customary coping mechanisms, whether or not these mechanisms in themselves are adaptive or maladaptive. Failure of the coping mechanisms brings about a state of unrest, confusion, pain, and panic which incapacitates the individual to some degree. He appears to be in a box from which he cannot escape no matter how hard he tries. He is against the proverbial brick wall. The result of being in a painful situation in which one seems unable to either fight back or run away is a severe increase in the level of anxiety.

It is at this point, when customary stress mechanisms have failed, that the individual is likely to try new approaches and is the most amenable to changing his behavior. If new coping mechanisms fail or help is not available, the crisis situation may reach a state of panic in which destructive behavior will occur.

The crisis cycle may be diagrammed as shown on page 196. Diagram 1 illustrates the successful resolution of a simple crisis situation. Diagram 2 illustrates a severe, more complex crisis situation which was resolved in a positive manner in that new learning has occurred and the crisis is ameliorated. It is possible, however, that the new coping mechanisms and the resolution are both maladaptive and may bring about future crises. The immediate crisis, however, will have been resolved. Diagram 3 illustrates failure in the crisis situation with destruction as a result.

CODE: S=Stress   A=Anxiety   C=Coping Behavior   W=Waiting Period
         <=Greater   F=Failure   R=Positive Resolution

DIAGRAM 1

$$S \longrightarrow A \longrightarrow C \longrightarrow W \longrightarrow R$$

DIAGRAM 2

$$S \longrightarrow A \longrightarrow C \longrightarrow W \longrightarrow F \longrightarrow <S \longrightarrow <A \longrightarrow New\ C \longrightarrow R$$

DIAGRAM 3

$$S \rightarrow A \rightarrow C \rightarrow W \rightarrow F \rightarrow (<S \rightarrow <A \rightarrow New\ C \rightarrow F) \rightarrow Destruction$$

Types of Crisis Resolution

Crisis situations must be resolved. Positive resolution may consist of acceptance or active resignation to a situation which cannot be changed, such as the death of a loved one. Resolution also may occur as the result of learning new coping mechanisms. If the learning and coping mechanisms are adaptive in nature the resolution will effectually teach the individual how to deal with future crises. If the learning is maladaptive, future crises are likely to be resolved in a maladaptive manner. For example, an individual is hungry and without money. That is a crisis! He may obtain a job that will provide the money. That is a positive resolution. The crisis has been solved and he has learned a useful skill. However, he may decide to steal to obtain the money. Stealing will resolve the immediate money-food crisis but may result in continued stealing which is not only a maladaptive societal response but is also likely to result in a future crisis.

Finally, the crisis may be resolved, or at least ended, by the physical or psychological destruction of the self, physical destruction by suicide, psychological destruction by total apathy or psychosis.

Crisis accompanies change in customary behaviors if they are altered. Most people are well aware of the discomfort arising from "getting out of a rut." The "rut" may be uncomfortable but at least one has learned how to live in it. Getting out means changing many aspects of one's behavior, attitudes, emotions, and thinking.

The individual begins to learn how to cope with stress as he matures. Most mothers are aware of their child's progress from one developmental level to another by the amount of stress they observe in both the child and themselves. This type of stress is developmental and is the school in which one learns coping behavior which prepares the individual to deal not only with developmental stress but also with stress arising from external sources.

The concern of this workbook in crisis intervention is primarily with developmental stress, since the implementation of the nursing care plan is considered a learning or developmental process. The implementation of the care plan will, therefore, be accompanied by major or minor crises. A crisis situation will also exist in the milieu because change in the client also requires change in others and in the milieu. If the nursing care plan is to be implemented successfully, the nurse needs to recognize a crisis situation and be able to help the client resolve the crisis in an adaptive manner.

The most important clue to the existence of a crisis is the level of anxiety observed either in the client or in others with whom he interacts. Heightened anxiety is to be expected as implementation begins, but when it reaches the proportions at which the nurse observes the client distorting reality or unable to focus on the problem, his anxiety level is too severe to warrant maintaining it at that level.

If the crisis is subacute, symptomatology may be masked and the anxiety indicative of crisis will be expressed in a variety of ways such as unrealistic complaining, physical complaints, physical tension, excessive discouragement, and exacerbation or exaggeration of psychological problems.

Steps in Crisis Intervention

The first step in crisis intervention is to *evaluate the degree of risk* involved. If the nurse considers the situation life-threatening, she should immediately secure whatever assistance is available to her. The crises involved in implementing a nursing care plan may become intense but ordinarily they are not life-threatening. It is the subacute crisis that is being considered in this workbook. The risk involved in the subacute crisis is that the client, experiencing stress or failure, may refuse to continue with the implementation of the care plan.

At the first indication that the situation is reaching crisis proportions, the nurse needs to defuse the situation. Defusing may consist of physical removal from the situation causing the crisis or of psychological measures usually referred to as "talking down" which allows a release of pent up energy. For example, the client who has a phobia about crowds and who embarks on a desensitization program with the nurse may panic as he makes his first attempt to enter a supermarket, even with the nurse at his side. In this instance, the situation may be defused by physical removal from the supermarket.

An example of psychological defusing exists when the client who has difficulty in initiating social interactions without hostility vituperously attacks members of the group in which he is involved. To defuse the situation the nurse may calmly discuss with the client within the group situation the behavior that she is observing. Reflecting to the client that he is expressing angry feelings whose source needs to be discussed within the group setting may decrease his anxiety enough by her indication of concern for him that he may be able to assess his behavior.

"Talking-down" is most likely to be an after the fact event in a nurse-client relationship. The client enters the interview situation in an obvious state of stress. With or without encouragement he may proceed to tell the nurse how and why he is anxious. The act of sharing his experiences and feelings usually defuses the immediate crisis, and nurse and client can move to the next step in crisis intervention. The client's anxiety must be at the level where he is able to attend, respond, and recollect with a reasonable amount of clarity and reality.

The second step consists of *determining and assessing the actual cause of the crisis.* In implementing the plan of care, hopefully the nurse has prepared the client for stress and failure as a part of change. Knowing that these are to be expected and are not indicative of total failure, the client can recall data which presented the crisis-causing problem. His observations may result in a modification of the care plan, but may also simply mean that he has a need for encouragement to continue as planned realizing that he is learning to tolerate stress. Obviously, if the cause of the stress is unrelated to the care plan, the nurse and client are facing a situation which may require the postponement of the care plan until a more favorable period. The nurse may be in a position to assist with the added crisis or she may find it necessary to refer the client to other professionals.

The third step in crisis intervention closely follows assessment of the cause. If modification of the care plan is required, then a *plan of intervention must be developed* that will encompass those difficulties presenting the crisis. If, on the other hand, the client is in need of encouragement to continue his progress, then the nurse will indicate to the client the reasons for his anxiety and help him develop toleration and control of his emotions. The third step, then, is to develop a plan to intervene in the crisis consistent with its cause.

A common problem lies in the fact that in beginning a behavioral change, the client looks at a far distant goal and all of the suffering and work involved. Discouragement at the prospect of a monumental task quickly follows. When the client expresses such discouragement, it is helpful to help him define an immediate rather than a long-range goal, one in which he is likely to experience success. *Breaking large problems into smaller, clearly defined areas* which can be achieved with relative ease usually helps dissipate the discouragement and relieves the crisis. For example, a freshman college student who thinks of four years of work, study, papers, projects, exams, and reading is likely to be very discouraged. If he breaks his problem down into small segments, such as getting through the first semester or even writing the first paper, he not only may find the prospect less dismal but may even find some enjoyment involved.

Once a plan of intervention is made, the client and the nurse need to explore methods by which the intervention can be completed. Care must be taken to maintain consistency with the overall nursing care plan and not just to relieve the immediate crisis. The *determination of the method of intervention* consists of the fifth step in crisis intervention.

Hopefully, the sixth step, that of *positive resolution,* completes the intervention. As stated earlier, resolution does not necessarily mean that the crisis "goes away." It may mean that the crisis situation is resolved by active resignation to the situation by the client. For example, sudden awareness that one is sixty-five years of age and must retire tomorrow is a crisis which will not "go away." Never again will one be twenty! Acceptance of the aging process is the resolution of crisis. Positive resolution invariably results in some new learning. Changes in coping behavior, new attitudes, new skills, all come as a result of some crisis. Knowing this, the nurse need not fear that the crisis will destroy her client but rather she will welcome the crisis as an opportunity for the client to grow and mature in an adaptive manner with her guidance.

Resolution should be accompanied by evaluation of what happened, why it happened, and how to handle a crisis so that in the future, when the client faces stress independently, he will have gained understanding not only of what to expect but also of what to do about it and when and where to seek help. There is no one who does not at some time need the concerned help of others. There is no one who never faces a crisis.

GUIDE FOR CRISIS INTERVENTION

Directions: Complete the following items using data from your process recordings and your experience.

1. As implementation of the care plan begins or progresses, describe signs of increased anxiety. Include an assessment of the level of anxiety.

2. Describe coping mechanisms being used as to:
   a. Technical name:

   b. Adaptive characteristics:

   c. Maladaptive characteristics:

   d. Results of coping behavior:

   e. Example of new coping behavior:

f.   Example of usual coping behavior:

g.   Reappearance of discarded coping behavior:

3.   Indicate the approximate length of the waiting period between the use of coping behavior and the results of the coping behavior. Describe the client's behavior during the waiting period and his tolerance for the waiting.

4.   Describe behavior that caused you to think that the client was in a crisis situation.

5.   Using the code on page 196, diagram the crisis situation.

6. Using the steps outlined in the workbook, describe your crisis interventions. Include the client's responses.

Step 1

Step 2

Step 3

Step 4

Step 5

Step 6

7. Describe the reactions of others in the milieu who customarily interact with the client.

8. Describe the reactions of others to your attempts at crisis intervention.

9. Describe the quality and quantity of assistance offered by others to you and the client during the crisis intervention.

10. Describe the reactions of others to the final resolution.

11. Describe new learning by your client that has occurred as a result of the crisis.

12. Describe the client's evaluation of the resolution of the crisis. Include any differences between your evaluation and the client's, reasons for the differences, and need to resolve the disparity between the two evaluations.

INSTRUCTOR'S COMMENTS

CHAPTER 16

Termination

The end of any relationship or experience inevitably brings with it a sense of loss. All of us know the sorrow that comes with parting from familiar friends and places. The deeper the personal involvement, the greater will be the loss experienced. Erich Lindemann describes certain behaviors normally following loss and some pathological reactions to grief.[1] The most common symptoms of normal grief as he describes them are:

1. Somatic symptoms such as anorexia, fatigue, and inability to sleep.
2. Preoccupation with the image of the deceased.
3. Feelings of guilt.
4. Feelings of hostility.
5. Loss of patterns of conduct.

Lindemann claims that pathological symptoms are primarily the result of a denial of the loss.

The reaction of both client and nurse to the termination of the nurse-client relationship is a grief reaction in which the symptoms of loss will be noted in proportion to the involvement each feels. The impending separation will also reactivate feelings of grief that have occurred with other separations. Sometimes it is the knowledge of the grief that comes with loss that prevents the patient from becoming involved in any close relationship.

The nurse attempts to help her client in advance to start the grief work. Her objectives are to help him avoid a denial of the impending loss and express the feelings of guilt and hostility.

The process of termination actually was started when the date of the final meeting was announced during the orientation period. At that time, however, to both student and client, termination appeared a long way off. Therefore, the nurse reminds the client again of the closing date a few weeks in advance of the final meeting, depending of course, on the time allotted to the entire relationship. In this way she starts the grief work in time to help both herself and the client tolerate the loss.

---

[1] Lindemann, Erich: "Symptomatology and Management of Acute Grief." *American Journal of Psychiatry*, Vol. 101, No. 2, Sept. 1944.

Perhaps the best way the nurse can understand the client's reaction to termination is to remember how she herself felt on similar occasions, such as when she first left home. She may also cast a critical eye on the way she is feeling and behaving as the termination approaches. Many students at this time will display hostility through excessive questioning not only of the value of their work but the necessity of their having been assigned such a task anyway. They will find much fault with the quality and quantity of the supervisory help they received, will complain about the psychiatric unit, the personnel involved, and, in fact, anything else that occurs to them. Perhaps the most prominent feature is the terrible feeling of guilt that arises from the thought that she is abandoning the patient. The client meanwhile is likely to feel that he is, in fact, being abandoned and will convey this idea to the nurse by his behavior.

The activities of the client may affect the nurse's feelings of guilt so that she may have difficulty in completing the termination. Attempts by the client to insure the continuation of the relationship beyond the date set for its completion are common. Fantasies about the return of the nurse may also occur. To combat such unrealistic thoughts, the nurse needs to understand the effect of her own feelings, particularly of guilt, so that she is not tempted to prolong termination. Adhering to the termination date as stated helps the patient perceive the reality of the loss. It also allows him to start and complete the grief work knowing that there is no alternative—the nurse will not return.

Many times when termination is started, the client considers that he is about to be rejected. Rather than allowing himself to be cast aside, he may prefer to take control of the situation by refusing to see or talk with the nurse. In this way, he himself terminates the relationship, rejecting the nurse before she can reject him.

Perhaps the hostility and guilt of the client are easier for the nurse to bear than the sight of him apparently regressing to the same level of functioning as when the relationship began. If the nurse has started the termination process early enough, she may be successful in helping the client limit his regression so that eventually he may again reach the point achieved during the nurse-client relationship. The fact that the nurse is able to help the client avoid denial, suitably express feelings of guilt and hostility, and tolerate the reality of the loss is in itself a valuable experience in the art of adaptive living.

Termination involves evaluation. The nurse attempts to help the client assess the progress he has made. He assesses what changes occurred, why they occurred, the effects on himself and others of the changes made, and how he may maintain and continue his progress.

Part of his assessment will include the understanding of the values of human relationships. This means that he will need to know not only what the nurse has meant to him, but also what he has meant to the nurse. The nurse needs, therefore, to indicate her feelings about termination. There is no intention to suggest that termination is either a mutual admiration party or a mutual wailing session. Without losing professional status the nurse can indicate that she feels sad at the termination, that the relationship has been important to her, and that she realizes the client also feels sad. In discussing past events, both the pleasant and unpleasant, she helps to put the relationship into perspective. All relationships end at sometime, but the value of the relationship does not diminish. The final lesson of the nurse-client relationship.is completed as the client accepts the sorrow of loss but is ready to live again.

GUIDE FOR TERMINATION OF NURSE-CLIENT RELATIONSHIP

Directions: Discuss the following questions and then plan your termination procedure. Complete the items in the guide from your interaction notes.

Questions for Discussion before the Final Interview

1. What does the client need to know about the termination of the interviews? When does he need this information? Why does he need it?

2. What problems do you expect the client will have with ending the interview? What means are available to him to express his problems?

3. What kinds of information do you wish to include in the terminating interview? Why?

4. What problems will you have with yourself when ending the nurse-client relationship?

Information about Termination

1. What did you tell the client about terminating the interview?

2. How many times did you give information about terminating? When did you give this information?

3. What indications did the client give that he understood or did not understand the information?

4. What indications did the client give that he remembered the information?

Response to Termination

1. What was the client's response to the information about termination the first time you gave it? The second time? Other times? At the final interview?

2. Describe symptoms of loss observed in your client. Describe your intervention and its results. Evaluate it.

3. Describe any symptoms you have observed which indicate that your client is denying the termination.

    a. Describe your intervention and its results, and evaluate it.

4.   Describe any means the client used to try to maintain the relationship beyond the stated date of termination. Indicate your intervention, the results of the intervention, and the evaluation of your action.

5.   Describe any regression that the client displayed.

a.   Describe steps you took to limit the regression. Include the results of your intervention. Evaluate your activity.

6.   What defense mechanism other than denial did the client use to help himself deal with the anxiety of separation?

7.   How did you feel about giving the information concerning termination? What did you do about your feelings? What will you do tomorrow about your feelings of separation?

Assessment of the Relationship

1. Describe what the client assesses as having been of the greatest value to him.

2. Describe what the client assesses as having been of least value.

3. Describe the client's evaluation of a nurse-client relationship. Have his values changed in this respect from what they were in the beginning?

4. List any statements that indicate he equates this termination with past losses. Include any general remarks he makes about relationships having to end.

5. Describe your evaluation of the relationship as you presented it to the client. Include his response to your evaluation.

6. List any statements you made concerning your own emotions at termination. Include the client's response.

7. Was the experience worthwhile to you?

INSTRUCTOR'S COMMENTS

PART IV

EVALUATION

CHAPTER 17

Descriptive Data

Evaluation is a procedure followed throughout the nurse-client relationship to enable the nurse to conduct her activities in a purposeful and therapeutic manner. A final evaluation gives her a comprehensive view of her client, his progress, and that which encouraged or impeded progress. It helps establish guidelines for future nursing activity as it provides an experimental basis to complement the theoretical background already acquired.

The final evaluation is presented in three sections. The first section (the present chapter) is descriptive and is designed to compare the mental health status of the client during the orientation, working, and termination stages. The second section (Chapter 18) is an assessment of the learning acquired by the client using Hewett's steps in the learning process as a base. The third section (Chapter 19) is an assessment of the learning acquired by the nurse, based on Hewett's approach.

Review the various guides to obtain the necessary data.

Directions: Complete the following assessments from data in previous guides, your recordings, and your observations.

Viewpoint	Orientation	Working Phase	Termination
Image of Self			
Image of Others			
Image of Environment			

Describe an experience in which one of the changes you have indicated on page 216 took place.

1.   Review the guides to determine the emotions expressed by the patient. Did the patient express emotions at the close of the nurse-client relationship that he did not express in the beginning? List changes in quantity, quality, and appropriateness of emotions expressed as you observed them when you first began the nurse-client relationship, again during the working phase, and finally at the termination period. (See the form on page 218 for listing these emotions.)

Describe an experience in which the client expressed emotion appropriately.

2.   Review the guides to determine the client's ability to communicate with you at the beginning of the relationship, during the working phase, and finally during the termination period. (See form on page 219 for this review.)

3.   Review the guides to determine the developmental levels at which the client functioned in the beginning, during working phase, and at termination. Describe one experience which indicated movement from one developmental level to another. (See form on page 220 for this review.)

Time	Emotion	Quality	Quantity	Appropriateness
Orientation				
Working Phase				
Termination				
Orientation	Emotion			
Working Phase				
Termination				
Orientation	Emotion			
Working Phase				
Termination				

Communication Usage	Orientation	Working Phase	Termination
Neologisms			
Loose Association			
Circumstantiality			
Indefinite Words			
Concrete Terminology			
Abstract Terminology			
Ability to Describe			
Ability to Clarify			

Ability to Function	Orientation	Working Phase	Termination
Trust			
Autonomy			
Self Identification			
Industry			
Creativity			
Interpersonal Relations			
Interdependence			

INSTRUCTOR'S COMMENTS

CHAPTER 18

Assessment of the Client's Learning

Directions: Using data from the working or from the terminal phases of the relationship, complete the following assessment. Limit the assessment of learning to the implementation of the goals of the care plan. Some learning will have occurred during the orientation period, but the assessment is directed toward that which is a direct result of the agreement between nurse and client as to the area of behavioral learning to be developed. Some space is provided in which the nurse will indicate areas toward which the client may direct change in the future.

Attending Skills

Phase	Problem	Effect of Problem	Intervention	Response to Intervention
Working				
Terminal				
Future Changes Indicated			Suggested Intervention	

Responding Skills

Phase	Problem	Effect of Problem	Intervention	Response to Intervention
Working				
Terminal				
Future Changes Indicated		Suggested Intervention		

Exploratory Skills

Phase	Problem	Effect of Problem	Intervention	Response to Intervention
Working				
Terminal				
Future Changes Indicated			Suggested Intervention	

Social Skills

Phase	Problem	Effect of Problem	Intervention	Response to Intervention
Working				
Terminal				
Future Changes Indicated			Suggested Intervention	

Mastery

Phase	Problem	Effect of Problem	Intervention	Response to Intervention
Working				
Terminal				
Areas of Problem Incompletely Mastered			Resources available to client to complete mastery of problem	Method taken to encourage use of resources for completion of mastery

INSTRUCTOR'S COMMENTS

CHAPTER 19

Assessment of the Nurse's Learning

The assessment guides require the nurse to assess her learning during each of the stages of the nurse-client relationship. Each guide indicates the specific learning dimension to be assessed, e.g., attending, responding, exploratory, social, and mastery. In assessing mastery skills the nurse is expected to assess her ability to complete mastery of the skills unique to the various stages of the relationship. For example, during the orientation period she assesses her ability to observe, report, and interpret data. During the working phase she assesses her ability to develop and implement a nursing care plan, including her reasons for selecting a particular theoretical framework as a base. During the terminal period she assesses her ability to complete the grief work required for both herself and her client.

Directions: Using data from your instructor's comments, comments of your client, comments from your peers, and your own observations of behavior throughout the course of the nurse-client relationship, complete the assessment tool on pages 232 to 236.

Attending Skills

Phase	Problem	Effect of Problem	Steps Taken to Correct Problem
Orientation			
Working			
Terminal			
Future Changes Indicated			

Responding Skills

Phase	Problem	Effect of Problem	Steps Taken to Correct Problem
Orientation			
Working			
Terminal			
Future Changes Indicated			

Exploratory Skills

Phase	Problem	Effect of Problem	Steps Taken to Correct Problem
Orientation			
Working			
Terminal			
Future Changes Indicated			

Social Skills

Phase	Problem	Effect of Problem	Steps Taken to Correct Problem
Orientation			
Working			
Terminal			
Future Changes Indicated			

Mastery

Phase	Problem	Effect of Problem	Steps Taken to Correct Problem
Orientation			
Working			
Terminal			
Future Changes Indicated			

SUMMATION

1. Describe the major learning you acquired from this nurse-client relationship.

2. List knowledge you needed but did not have at the appropriate time.

3. What helped you most in establishing your nurse-client relationship?

4. What prevented or hindered you in reaching your goals?

5. How do you justify your nursing intervention if your client has regressed to a developmental level that is earlier than that at which he functioned when you began your interaction?

INSTRUCTOR'S COMMENTS

Bibliography

General

1. Adelson, Daniel and Kalis, Betty L.: *Community Psychology and Mental Health.*
   Scranton, Pennsylvania: Chandler Publishing Co., 1970.
2. Allport, Gordon W.: *Becoming: Basic Considerations for a Psychology of Personality.*
   New Haven: Yale University Press, 1955.
3. Anderson, Camilla: *Beyond Freud.* New York: Harper Brothers, 1957.
4. Arieti, Silvano: *Interpretation of Schizophrenia.* New York: Robert Brunner, Inc.,
   1955.
5. Arieti, Silvano: *The Will to be Human.* New York: Quadrangle Books, 1972.
6. Arieti, Silvano: *American Handbook of Psychiatry, 2nd edition, Vols. I, II, and III.*
   New York: Basic Books, 1974.
7. Artiss, Kenneth I., Ed.: *The Symptom as Communication in Schizophrenia.* New York:
   Grune and Stratton, 1959.
8. Bandura, A. and Walters, R. H.: *Social Learning and Personality Development.*
   New York: Holt, Rinehart and Winston, 1963.
9. Barnlund, Dean C.: *Interpersonal Communication: Survey and Studies.* Boston:
   Houghton Mifflin Co., 1968.
10. Beier, Ernst: *The Silent Language of Psychotherapy.* Chicago: Aldine Publishing Co.,
    1967.
11. Berne, Eric: *Games People Play.* New York: Grove Press Inc., 1964.
12. Bertocci, Peter and Millard, Richard: *Personality and the Good.* New York: David
    McKay Co., 1963.
13. Birney, Robert and Teevan, Richard, Eds.: *Measuring Human Motivation.* Princeton:
    Van Nostrand Co., 1962.
14. Brody, Eugene B. and Redlich, Frederick C.: *Psychotherapy with Schizophrenics.*
    New York: International Universities Press Inc., 1952.
15. Brown, R.: *Social Psychology.* New York: The Free Press, 1965.
16. Bruch, Hilde: *Learning Psychotherapy.* Cambridge, Massachusetts: Harvard University
    Press, 1974.
17. Cameron, Norman: *Personality Development and Psychopathology.* Boston: Houghton
    Mifflin Co., 1963.
18. Carkhuff, Robert: *The Art of Helping.* Amherst, Massachusetts: Human Resources
    Development Press, 1972.
19. Carkhuff, Robert: *The Art of Problem Solving.* Amherst, Massachusetts: Human
    Resources Development Press, 1972.

241

20. Clarizio, Harvey, Ed.: *Mental Health and the Educational Process*. Chicago: Rand McNally and Co., 1969.

21. Clarizio, Harvey and McCoy, George F.: *Behavior Disorders in School-Aged Children*. Scranton, Ohio: Chandler Publishing Co., 1970.

22. Clark, Donald H., Ed.: *Psychology of Education*. New York: The Free Press, 1967.

23. Corsini, Raymond J., Ed.: *Current Psychotherapies*. Itasca, Illinois: F. T. Peacock Publishers Inc., 1973.

24. Cowen, Emory. Ed. by Gardner, Elmer and Zax, Melvin: *Emergent Approaches to Mental Health Problems*. New York: Appleton-Century-Crofts, 1967.

25. Daniel, Robert, Ed.: *Contemporary Readings in General Psychology*. Boston: Houghton Mifflin Co., 1959.

26. Davis, Murray: *Intimate Relations*. New York: The Free Press, 1975.

27. Deese, James and Hulse, Stewart: *Psychology of Learning*. New York: McGraw-Hill Co., 1967.

28. Dreger, Ralph: *Fundamentals of Personality*. Philadelphia: J. B. Lippincott, 1962.

29. Erikson, Erik: *Childhood and Society*. New York: W. W. Norton Co., 1950.

30. Eysenck, H. J.: *Behavior Therapy and the Neuroses*. New York: Pergamon Press, 1960.

31. Frank, Jerome D.: *Persuasion and Healing,* 2nd edition. Baltimore: Johns-Hopkins University Press, 1973.

32. Frankl, Viktor: *Man's Search for Meaning*. Boston: Beacon Press, 1959.

33. Freud, Sigmund: *A general Introduction to Psychoanalysis*. New York: Washington Square Press, 1963.

34. Galvin, Kathleen M. and Book, Cassandra: *Speech-Communication*. Skokie, Illinois: Nat'l Textbook Co., 1972.

35. Garrett, Annette: *Interviewing: Its Principles and Methods*. New York: Family Service Assn. of America, 1972.

36. Goffman, Erving: *Presentation of Self in Everyday Life*. Woodstock, New York: Overlook Press, 1974.

37. Greene, Hannah: *I Never Promised You a Rose Garden*. New York: Holt, Rinehart and Winston, 1964.

38. Haber, Ralph, Ed.: *Current Research in Motivation*. New York: Holt, Rinehart and Winston, 1966.

39. Hall, John: *The Psychology of Learning*. Philadelphia: J. B. Lippincott, 1966.

40. Harris, Irving: *Emotional Blocks to Learning*. New York: Free Press of Glencoe, 1961.

41. Harris, M.: *The Nature of Cultural Things*. New York: Random House Inc., 1964.

42. Harris, Thomas: *I'm O.K. — Your're O.K.* New York: Avon Books, 1973.

43. Hewett, Frank: *Emotionally-disturbed Child in the Classroom*. Boston: Allyn Bacon Co., 1968.

44. Hewett, Frank and Forness, Steven: *Education of Exceptional Learners*. Boston: Allyn Bacon Co., 1974.

45. Hilgard, Ernest and Atkinson, Richard: *Introduction to Psychology*. 4th edition. New York: Harcourt, Brace and World Inc., 1967.

46. Holt, John: *How Children Fail*. New York: Dell Publishing Co., Inc., 1972.

47. Jackson, Don, Ed.: *The Etiology of Schizophrenia*. New York: Basic Books Inc., 1960.

48. Jahoda, Marie: *Current Concepts of Positive Mental Health*. New York: Basic Books Inc., 1960.

49. James, Muriel and Jongeward, Dorothy: *Born to Win*. Reading, Massachusetts: Addison-Wesley Publishing Co., 1971.

50. Jones, Maxwell: *Beyond the Therapeutic Community*. New Haven: Yale University Press, 1972.

51. Kadushin, Alfred: *The Social Work Interview*. New York: Columbia University Press, 1972.

52. Kahn, J. H.: *Human Growth and the Development of Personality*. New York: Pergamon Press, 1965.

53. Kantor, David and Lehr, William: *Inside the Family.* San Francisco: Jossey-Bass Inc., Publishers, 1975.
54. Kephart, W.: *Family, Society and the Individual.* Boston: Houghton Mifflin Co., 1961.
55. Kessler, Jane: *Psychopathology of Childhood.* Englewood Cliffs, New Jersey: Prentice-Hall, 1966.
56. Knapp, Peter, Ed.: *Expression of the Emotions in Man.* New York: International Universities Press, 1963.
57. Krasner, L. and Ullman, L. P.: *Research in Behavior Modification.* New York: Holt, Rinehart and Winston, 1965.
58. Kroeber, T. C.: "The Coping Functions of the Ego Mechanisms," in White, R. W., Ed., *The Study of Lives.* New York: Atherton Press, 1963.
59. Krumboltz, John and Thorsen, Carl: *Behavioral Counseling.* New York: Holt, Rinehart and Winston, 1969.
60. Laing, R. D.: *The Politics of Experience.* New York: Random House, 1967.
61. Laing, R. D.: *Knots.* New York: Random House, 1968.
62. Laing, R. D.: *The Divided Self.* New York: Random House, 1969.
63. Langner, T. S. and Michael, S. T.: *Life, Stress and Mental Health.* New York: Free Press of Glencoe, 1963.
64. Lawrence, D. H. and Festinger, L.: *Deterrents and Reinforcement.* Stanford: Stanford University Press, 1962.
65. Lidz, Theodore: *The Origin and Treatment of Schizophrenic Disorders.* New York: Basic Books, 1973.
66. Lieb, Julian, Lipsitch, Ian and Slaby, Andrea: *The Crisis Team.* Hagerstown, Maryland: Harper and Row, 1973.
67. Lindgren, Henry: *Psychology of Personal Development.* New York: American Books, 1964.
68. MacKinnon, Roger and Michels, Robert: *The Psychiatric Interview in Clinical Practice.* Philadelphia: W. B. Saunders Co., 1971.
69. Madigan, Marian: *Psychology, Principles and Applications.* St. Louis: C. V. Mosby Co., 1962.
70. Martin, Lealone: *Mental Health/Mental Illness.* New York: McGraw-Hill Co., 1970.
71. Maslow, Abraham: *Motivation and Personality.* New York: Harper Brothers, 1954.
72. Maslow, Abraham: *New Knowledge in Human Values.* New York: Harper Brothers, 1959.
73. May, Rollo: *The Meaning of Anxiety.* New York: The Ronald Press, 1950.
74. May, Rollo, Ed.: *Existential Psychology.* New York: Random House, 1961.
75. May, Rollo, Angel, Ernest and Ellenberger, Henri F., Eds.: *Existence.* New York: Simon and Schuster, 1967.
76. Mendelson, Myer: *Psychoanalytic Concepts of Depression.* 2nd edition. New York: Halsted Press, 1974.
77. Menninger, Karl and Holzman, Philip: *Theory of Psychoanalytic Technique.* 2nd edition. New York: Basic Books, 1973.
78. Menolascino, Frank: *Psychiatric Approaches to Mental Retardation.* New York: Basic Books, 1970.
79. Milton, Ohmer, Ed.: *Behavior Disorders: Perspectives and Trends.* Philadelphia: J. B. Lippincott, 1965.
80. Morgan, Clifford: *Introduction to Psychology.* New York: McGraw-Hill Co., 1961.
81. Mowrer, O. Hobart: *Learning Theory and Behavior.* New York: John Wiley and Sons, 1960.
82. Murray, Edward: *Motivation and Emotion.* New York: Appleton-Century-Crofts, 1965.
83. Nathan, Peter and Harris, Sandra: *Psychopathology and Society.* New York: McGraw-Hill Co., 1975.
84. Newcomb, T. M., Converse, P. E. and Turner, R. H.: *Social Psychology.* New York: Holt, Rinehart and Winston, 1964.

85. Noyes, Arthur and Kolb, Lawrence: *Modern Clinical Psychiatry.* Philadelphia: W. B. Saunders Co., 1963.
86. Parker, Beulah: *My Language Is Me.* New York: Basic Books Inc., 1962.
87. Rabkin, Richard: *Inner and Outer Space.* New York: W. W. Norton Co., 1970.
88. Reich, Theodore: *Listening With the Third Ear.* New York: Farrar, Straus, 1948.
89. Rogers, Carl R.: *Client-Centered Therapy.* Boston: Houghton Mifflin Co., 1951.
90. Rogers, Carl R.: *On Becoming a Person.* Boston: Houghton Mifflin Co., 1961.
91. Rosenbaum, Peter and Beebe, John E., III: *Psychiatric Treatment: Crisis/Clinic/Consultation.* New York: McGraw-Hill Co., 1975.
92. Ruesch, Jurgen and Bateson, Gregory: *Communication: The Social Matrix of Psychiatry.* New York: W. W. Norton Co., 1951.
93. Ruesch, Jurgen: *Therapeutic Communication.* New York: W. W. Norton Co., 1961.
94. Schaefer, Halmuth and Martin, Patrick: *Behavior Therapy.* New York: McGraw-Hill Co., 1975.
95. Sechehaye, Marguerite: *Autobiography of a Schizophrenic Girl.* New York: Grune and Stratton Co., 1951.
96. Sechehaye, Marguerite: *A New Psychotherapy in Schizophrenia.* New York: Grune and Stratton Co., 1956.
97. Sechrest, Lee and Wallace, John: *Psychology and Human Problems.* Columbus, Ohio: Charles E. Merrill Publishing Co., 1967.
98. Secord, P. F. and Bachman, C. W.: *Social Psychology.* New York: McGraw-Hill Co., 1964.
99. Silverstein, Max: *Psychiatric Aftercare.* Philadelphia: University of Pennsylvania Press, 1968.
100. Simon, Sidney B.: *Values Clarification.* New York: Hart Publishing Co., 1972.
101. Speck, Ross and Attneave, Carol: *Family Networks.* New York: Random House, 1973.
102. Spiegel, John: *Transactions: The Interplay Between Individual, Family, and Society.* New York: Aronson, 1971.
103. Spielberger, Charles, Ed.: *Anxiety and Behavior.* New York: Academic Press, 1966.
104. Stacey, C. L. and DeMartino, M. F., Eds.: *Understanding Human Motivation.* Cleveland: World Publishing Co., 1963.
105. Sullivan, Harry S.: *Interpersonal Theory of Psychiatry.* New York: W. W. Norton Co., 1953.
106. Sullivan, Harry S.: *Clinical Studies in Psychiatry.* New York: W. W. Norton Co., 1956.
107. Symonds, Percival M.: *Dynamic Psychology.* New York: Appleton-Century-Crofts, 1957.
108. Wepman, J. and Heine, R. W.: *Concepts of Personality.* Chicago: Aldine Publishing Co., 1963.
109. Wolman, Benjamin: *Success and Failure in Psychoanalysis and Psychotherapy.* New York: Macmillan Co., 1972.
110. Wrenn, Robert and Mencke, Reed: *Being: A Psychology of Self.* Chicago: Science Research Associates, 1975.

Nursing

1. Bermosk, L. S. and Murdane, M. J.: *Interviewing in Nursing.* 2nd edition. New York: Macmillan Co., 1973.
2. Bird, B.: *Talking with Patients.* Philadelphia: J. B. Lippincott, 1955.
3. Burd, Shirley F. and Marshall, Margaret, Eds.: *Some Clinical Approaches to Psychiatric Nursing.* New York: Macmillan Co., 1963.
4. Burgess, Ann and Lazare, Aaron: *Psychiatric Nursing in the Hospital and Community.* Englewood Cliffs, New Jersey: Prentice-Hall, 1973.
5. Burkhalter, Pamela: *Nursing Care of the Alcoholic and Drug Abuser.* New York: McGraw-Hill Co., 1975.

6. Burton, Genevive: *Development of Clinical Theory. Personal, Impersonal, and Inter-personal Relations.* 3rd edition. New York: Springer Publishing Co., 1970.
7. Fagin, Claire: *Family-Centered Nursing in Community Psychiatry.* Philadelphia: F. A. Davis Co., 1970.
8. Francis, Gloria and Munjas, Barbara: *Promoting Psychological Comfort.* Dubuque, Iowa: Wm. C. Brown Co., 1968.
9. Hays, Joyce and Larson, Kenneth: *Interacting With Patients.* New York: Macmillan Co., 1963.
10. Johnson, Margaret Anne: *Developing the Art of Understanding.* New York: Springer Publishing Co., 1967.
11. Kyes, Joan and Hofling, Charles: *Basic Psychiatric Concepts in Nursing.* Philadelphia: J. B. Lippincott Co., 1974.
12. Lockerby, Florence K.: *Communication for Nurses.* St. Louis: C. V. Mosby Co., 1963.
13. Maloney, Elizabeth: *Interpersonal Relations.* Dubuque, Iowa: Wm. C. Brown Co., 1966.
14. Manaser, J. C. and Werner, A. M.: *Instruments for Study of Nurse-Patient Interaction.* New York: Macmillan Co., 1964.
15. Matheney, Ruth and Topalis, Mary: *Psychiatric Nursing.* St. Louis: C. V. Mosby Co., 1974.
16. Mercer, Lianne and O'Conner, Patricia: *Fundamental Skills in the Nurse-Patient Relationship.* Philadelphia: W. B. Saunders, 1974.
17. Mereness, Dorothy and Taylor, Cecelia: *Essentials of Psychiatric Nursing.* 9th edition. St. Louis: C. V. Mosby Co., 1974.
18. Morgan, Arthur and Moreno, Judith: *The Practice of Mental Health Nursing: A Community Approach.* Philadelphia: J. B. Lippincott, 1973.
19. Muller, Theresa: *The Foundations of Human Behavior.* New York: G. P. Putnam's Sons, 1956.
20. Muller, Theresa: *Fundamentals of Psychiatric Nursing.* New Jersey: Littlefield, Adams, and Co., 1962.
21. Orlando, Ida Jean: *The Dynamic Nurse-Patient Relationship.* New York: G. P. Putnam's Sons, 1961.
22. Peplau, Hildegarde: *Interpersonal Relations in Psychiatric Nursing.* Philadelphia: J. B. Lippincott, 1960.
23. Peplau, Hildegarde: *Basic Principles of Patient Counseling.* 2nd edition. Philadelphia: Smith, Kline, and French Laboratories, 1964.
24. *Psychiatric Nursing 1946–1974: A Report on the State of the Art.* American Journal of Nursing Educational Services Division, New York, 1975.
25. Render, Helene and Weiss, M. Olga: *Nurse-Patient Relationships in Psychiatry.* 2nd edition. New York: McGraw-Hill Co., 1958.
26. Schwartz, Morris and Shockley, Emmy L.: *The Nurse and the Mental Patient.* New York: Russell Sage Foundation, 1956.
27. Tinkham, Catherine and Voorhies, Eleanor: *Community Health Nursing. Evolution and Process.* New York: Appleton-Century-Crofts, 1972.
28. Travelbee, Joyce: *Intervention in Psychiatric Nursing.* Philadelphia: F. A. Davis Co., 1970.
29. Travelbee, Joyce: *Interpersonal Aspects of Nursing.* 2nd edition. Philadelphia: F. A. Davis Co., 1971.
30. Ujhely, G. B.: *Determinants of the Nurse-Patient Relationship.* New York: Springer Publishing Co., 1968.
31. Vaillot, Sister Madeleine C.: *Commitment to Nursing.* Philadelphia: J. B. Lippincott, 1962.

Periodicals

1. Aguilera, D. C.: "Use of Physical Contact as a Technique of Non-Verbal Communication." ANA Reg. Clinical Conference, No. 4, 1965, 33-38.
2. Aguilera, D. C. and Messick, J. M.: "Crisis: The Psychiatric Nurse Intervenes." *Journal of Psychiatric Nursing,* May-June 1967, 5, 233-240.
3. Aiken, Linda and Aiken, J. L.: "A Systematic Approach to the Evaluation of Interpersonal Relations." *American Journal of Nursing,* May 1973, 73, 863-867.
4. Ambury, R. G.: "Crisis Intervention in Family and Adolescent Care." *Nursing Mirror,* Nov. 1972, 135, 33-36.
5. Barckley, Virginia: "The Nurse in Preventive Psychiatry." *Nursing Outlook,* May 1960, 8, 252-254.
6. Barron, F.: "An Ego-strength Scale Which Predicts Response to Psychotherapy." *Journal of Consulting Psychology,* 1953, 17, 327-333.
7. Berliner, A. K.: "The Two Milieus in Milieu Therapy." *Perspectives in Psychiatric Care,* Vol. 5, No. 6, 1967, 266-271.
8. Berlinger, B. S.: "Nursing a Patient in Crisis." *American Journal of Nursing,* Vol. 70, No. 10, Oct. 1970, 2154-2157.
9. Brown, F. G.: "Social Linkability," *American Journal of Nursing,* Vol. 71, No. 3, March 1971, 516-520.
10. Bucker, Kathleen: "The Treatment Role of the Psychiatric Nurse." *Perspectives in Psychiatric Care,* Vol. 4, No. 6, 1966, 15-19.
11. Bulbulyan, Ann et al: "Nurses in a Community Health Center." *American Journal of Nursing,* Vol. 69, No. 2, Feb. 1969, 328-331.
12. Christoffers, Carol A.: "An Existential Encounter." *Perspectives in Psychiatric Care,* Vol. 5, No. 4, 1967, 174-181.
13. Cleland, Virginia: "The Effects of Stress on Thinking." *American Journal of Nursing,* Vol. 67, No. 1, Jan. 1967, 108.
14. Cloud, E. D.: "The Plateau in Therapist-Patient Relationships." *Perspectives in Psychiatric Care,* Vol. 10, No. 3, 1973, 112-121.
15. Davis, A. J.: "Micro-ecology: Interactional Dimensions of Space." *Journal of Psychiatric Nursing,* Jan.-Feb. 1972, 10, 19-21.
16. Drucker, A. J. and Remmers, H. H.: "Environmental Determinants of Basic Difficulty Problems." *Journal of Abnormal and Social Psychology,* 1952, 47, 379-381.
17. Ehmann, V. E.: "Empathy: Its Origins, Characteristics and Process." *Perspectives in Psychiatric Care,* Vol. 9, No. 2, 1971, 72-80.
18. Fanning, V. L. et al.: "Patient Involvement in Planning Own Care." *Journal of Psychiatric Nursing,* Jan.-Feb. 1972, 10, 5-8.
19. Field, W. E. and Ruelke, Wylma: "Hallucinations and How to Deal with Them." *American Journal of Nursing,* Vol. 73, No. 4, April 1973, 638-640.
20. Flynn, G. E.: "The Nurse's Role: Interference or Intervention?" *Perspectives in Psychiatric Care,* Vol. 7, No. 4, 1969(b), 170-176.
21. Gregg, Dorothy: "Anxiety—A Factor in Nursing Care," *American Journal of Nursing,* Vol. 52, No. 2, Feb. 1952, 1363-1365.
22. Hargreaves, W. A. and Starkweather, F. H.: "Voice Quality in Depression." *Journal of Abnormal Psychology,* Vol. 70, No. 35, 1965, 218-220.
23. Hays, Dorothea R.: "Teaching a Concept of Anxiety to Patients." *Nursing Research,* Vol. 10, Spring, 1961.
24. Hitchcock, J. M.: "Crisis Intervention: The Pebble in the Pool." *American Journal of Nursing,* Vol. 73, No. 8, Aug. 1973, 1388-1390.
25. Holmes, Marguerite: "The Need to be Recognized." *American Journal of Nursing,* Vol. 61, No. 10, Oct. 1961, 88-87.
26. Ingraham, Blanche: "A Comprehensive Study of a Psychiatric Patient." *Persepectives in Psychiatric Care,* Vol. 2, No. 1, 1964, 22-30.

27. Ishiyama, Joaru, et al.: "Let's All Be Patients." *American Journal of Nursing,* Vol. 67, No. 3, March 1967, 569.
28. Jensen, Hellene and Tillotson, Gene: "Dependency in Nurse-Patient Relationship." *American Journal of Nursing,* Vol. 61, No. 5, May 1961, 76-81.
29. Kachelski, Audrey: "The Nurse-Patient Relationship." *American Journal of Nursing,* Vol. 61, No. 5, May 1961, 82-84.
30. Kalish, B. J.: "What Is Empathy?" *American Journal of Nursing,* Vol. 73, No. 9, Sept. 1973, 1548-1552.
31. Kalkman, M. E.: "Recognizing Emotional Problems." *American Journal of Nursing,* Vol. 68, No. 3, March 1968, 536-539.
32. King, J. M.: "The Initial Interview: Basis for Assessment in Crisis Intervention." *Perspectives in Psychiatric Care,* Vol. 5, No. 6, 1967, 256-261.
33. Kloes, K. B. and Weinberg, Ann: "Counter-transference: A Bilateral Phenomenon in a Learning Model." *Perspectives in Psychiatric Care,* Vol. 6, No. 4, 1968, 152-162.
34. Knicely, Kathryn: "The World of Disturbed Perception." *American Journal of Nursing,* Vol. 67, No. 5, May 1967, 998.
35. Kovace, Liberty W.: "A Therapeutic Relationship With a Patient and Family." *Perspectives in Psychiatric Care,* Vol. 4, No. 2, 1966, 11-21.
36. Kramer, E.: "Judgment of Personal Characteristics and Emotions from Nonverbal Properties of Speech." *Psychological Bulletin,* 1963, 60, 408-420.
37. Kramer, E.: "Elimination of Verbal Cues in Judgments of Emotion from Voice." *Journal of Abnormal and Social Psychology,* 1964, 68, 390-396.
38. Lovaas, O. I.: "Interaction between Verbal and Nonverbal Behavior." *Child Development,* 1961, 32, 329-336.
39. Maloney, E. M.: "The Subjective and Objective Definition of Crisis." *Perspectives in Psychiatric Care,* Vol. 9, No. 6, 1971, 257-268.
40. Masser, D.: "Communicating with a Schizophrenic Patient." *Perspectives in Psychiatric Care,* Vol. 8, No. 1, 1970, 36-38.
41. May, Rollo: "Existential Bases of Psychotherapy." *American Journal of Orthopsychiatry,* 1960, 30, 685-695.
42. Mayers, Marlene: "Home Visit — Ritual or Therapy?" *Nursing Outlook,* May 1973, 21, 328-331.
43. McElroy, Evelyn and Narciso, Anita: "Clinical Specialist in the Community Mental Health Program." *Journal of Psychiatric Nursing,* Jan.-Feb. 1971, 9, 19-26.
44. Mercer, Lianne: "Touch Comfort or Threat." *Perspectives in Psychiatric Care,* Vol. 4, No. 3, 1966, 20-25.
45. Moore, Judith: "The Dynamics of Schizophrenia." *Perspectives in Psychiatric Care,* Vol. 4, No. 5, 1966, 11-21.
46. Morris, K.: "Approach-Avoidance Conflict in the Orientation Phase of Therapy." (Abstract) *American Journal of Nursing,* Vol. 67, No. 12, Dec. 1967, 2586.
47. *National League for Nursing.* The League Exchange No. 26, Section A: Concepts in Nursing; Section B, Therapeutic Concepts.
48. Norris, Catherine: "Psychiatric Crises." *Perspectives in Psychiatric Care,* Vol. 5, No. 1, 1967, 21-28.
49. Parks, Suzanne L.: "Allowing Physical Distance as a Nursing Approach." *Perspectives in Psychiatric Care,* Vol. 4, No. 6, 1966, 31-35.
50. Peplau, Hildegarde: "Interpersonal Techniques. The Crux of Psychiatric Nursing." *American Journal of Nursing,* Vol. 62, No. 6, June 1962, 50.
51. Phillips, B. D.: "Terminating a Nurse-Patient Relationship." *American Journal of Nursing,* Vol. 68, No. 9, Sept. 1968, 1941-1942.
52. Renshaw, D. C.: "Psychiatric First Aid in an Emergency." *American Journal of Nursing,* Vol. 72, No. 3, March 1972, 497.
53. Repella, J. C.: "The Nurse, The Patient, The Environment, and Nursing Therapy." *Journal of Psychiatric Nursing,* Jan. 1963, 1, 16-20, 67-68.

54. Risley, Joan: "Nursing Intervention in Depression." *Perspectives in Psychiatric Care,* Vol. 5, No. 2, 1967, 65-75.

55. Robinson, A., Fried, M., Mallow, J., and Nuryean, P.: "The Role of the Nurse-Therapist in a Large Public Mental Hospital." *American Journal of Nursing,* Vol. 55, 1955, 55, 441.

56. Ryan, Betty Jane: "Teaching Self-expression." *Perspectives in Psychiatric Care,* Vol. 5, No. 4, 1967, 189-191.

57. Salerno, E. M.: "A Family in Crisis." *American Journal of Nursing,* Vol. 73, No. 1, Jan. 1973, 100-103.

58. Sene, B. S.: "Termination in the Student-Patient Relationship." *Perspectives in Psychiatric Care,* Vol. 7, No. 1, 1969, 39-45.

59. Shufer, Shirley.: "The Pediatric Mental Health Clinician." *Nursing Outlook,* Aug. 1971, 19, 543-545.

60. Sister Mary Michele Layton: "Behavior Therapy and Its Implications for Psychiatric Nursing." *Perspectives in Psychiatric Care,* Vol. 4, No. 2, 1966, 38-52.

61. Sister M. Rose Magdalen: "Depersonalization." *Perspectives in Psychiatric Care,* Vol. 1, No. 3, 1963, 29-31.

62. Stankiewicz, Barbara: "Guides to Nursing Intervention in the Projective Patterns of Suspicious Patients." *Perspectives in Psychiatric Care,* Vol. 2, No. 1, 1964, 39-45.

63. Stanko, Barbara: "Crisis Intervention After the Birth of a Defective Child." *Canadian Nurse,* July 1973, 69, 27-28.

64. Sugden, John: "Objectives in Psychiatric Nursing." *Nursing Times,* Oct. 1970, 66, 1297-1298.

65. Vennen, M. V.: "Notes on Termination." *Perspectives in Psychiatric Care,* Vol. 8, No. 5, 1970, 218-221.

66. Walker, L. O.: "Toward a Clearer Understanding of the Concept of Nursing Theory." *Nursing Research,* Sept.-Oct. 1971, 20, 428-435.

67. Williams, F.: "Intervention in Maturational Crises." *Perspectives in Psychiatric Care,* Vol. 9, No. 6, 1971, 240-246.

68. Wilson, D. C.: "A General Systems Approach to Attitude Therapy." *Hospital and Community Psychiatry,* Aug. 1970, 21, 264-267.

69. Wilson, H. S.: "Partners in Change." *American Journal of Nursing,* Vol. 71, No. 7, July 1971, 1400-1403.

70. Wolff, I. S.: "Acceptance." *American Journal of Nursing,* Vol. 72, No. 8, Aug. 1972, 1412-1415.